HANDBOOK OF
Good Psychiatric Management FOR
Borderline Personality Disorder
AND **Alcohol Use Disorder**

HANDBOOK OF
Good Psychiatric Management FOR
Borderline Personality Disorder
AND Alcohol Use Disorder

Edited by

Lois W. Choi-Kain, M.D., M.Ed.
Hilary S. Connery, M.D., Ph.D.

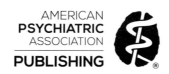

AMERICAN
PSYCHIATRIC
ASSOCIATION
PUBLISHING

If you wish to buy 50 or more copies of the same title, please go to www.appi.org/specialdiscounts for more information.

Copyright © 2025 American Psychiatric Association Publishing

ALL RIGHTS RESERVED

First Edition

Manufactured in the United States of America on acid-free paper
28 27 26 25 24   5 4 3 2 1

American Psychiatric Association Publishing
800 Maine Avenue SW, Suite 900
Washington, DC 20024–2812
www.appi.org

Library of Congress Cataloging-in-Publication Data
Names: Choi-Kain, Lois W, editor. | Connery, Hilary Smith, editor. |
  American Psychiatric Association Publishing, issuing body.
Title: Handbook of good psychiatric management for borderline personality
  disorder and alcohol use disorder / edited by Lois W. Choi-Kain, Hilary
  S. Connery.
Description: First edition. | Washington, DC : American Psychiatric
  Association Publishing, [2024] | Includes bibliographical references and
  index.
Identifiers: LCCN 2024019827 (print) | LCCN 2024019828 (ebook) | ISBN
  9781615375530 (paperback ; alk. paper) | ISBN 9781615375547 (ebook)
Subjects: MESH: Borderline Personality Disorder | Alcohol-Related Disorders
  | Comorbidity | Combined Modality Therapy--methods |
  Psychotherapy--methods
Classification: LCC RC569.5.B67 (print) | LCC RC569.5.B67 (ebook) | NLM
  WM 190.5.B5 | DDC 616.85/852--dc23/eng/20240719
LC record available at https://lccn.loc.gov/2024019827
LC ebook record available at https://lccn.loc.gov/2024019828

British Library Cataloguing in Publication Data
A CIP record is available from the British Library.

Dedication

*This book is dedicated to the memory of
Anne Osborn and Charlotte Watlington,
whose special spirit and sparkle shined bright
throughout their lives.
Despite the tenacious support of their families,
combined with efforts to get the best treatment
they could access, the challenges of
borderline personality and alcohol use disorder
could not be solved in time to keep them
here with us longer.*

*We learned from them that we must do better
to treat these disorders simultaneously.*

Contents

Lois W. Choi-Kain, M.D., M.Ed.
Hilary S. Connery, M.D., Ph.D.

Lois W. Choi-Kain, M.D., M.Ed.
Hilary S. Connery, M.D., Ph.D.

Marcelo J. A. A. Brañas, M.D.
Kimberley Siscoe, M.D.
Erik Ydrefelt, M.Sc. Psych
Marcos S. Croci, M.D.
Lois W. Choi-Kain, M.D., M.Ed.

Robert J. Gregory, M.D.
Lois W. Choi-Kain, M.D., M.Ed.

Rocco Iannucci, M.D.
Grace Murray, B.A.
Stephen Conway, M.D.

Daniel Price, M.D.
Erik Ydrefelt, M.Sc. Psych

Appendices

Contributors

Marcelo J. A. A. Brañas, M.D.
Co-Director, Adolescent Borderline Personality Disorder Outpatient Program, Institute of Psychiatry, University of São Paulo Medical School, São Paulo, Brazil

Lois W. Choi-Kain, M.D., M.Ed.
Director, Gunderson Personality Disorders Institute, Belmont, Massachusetts; Associate Professor, Harvard Medical School, Boston, Massachusetts

Hilary S. Connery, M.D., Ph.D.
Clinical Director, Division of Alcohol, Drugs, and Addiction, McLean Hospital, Belmont, Massachusetts; Assistant Professor of Psychiatry, Harvard Medical School, Boston, Massachusetts

Stephen Conway, M.D.
Consultation Liaison Psychiatry Fellow, Brigham and Women's Hospital, Harvard Medical School, Boston, Massachusetts

Marcos S. Croci, M.D.
Co-Director, Adolescent Borderline Personality Disorder Outpatient Program, Institute of Psychiatry, University of São Paulo Medical School, São Paulo, Brazil

Jeffrey DeVido, M.D., M.T.S.
Psychiatrist, MindTherapy Clinic; Assistant Clinical Professor, Psychiatry, University of California, San Francisco, School of Medicine, Weill Institute for Neurosciences, San Francisco, California

Carl Fleisher, M.D.
Co-Director and Medical Director, Boston Child Study Center,
Los Angeles, Los Angeles, California

Robin Gay, Ph.D.
Director of Psychological Services, Fernside Addiction Recovery
Program, McLean Hospital, Belmont, Massachusetts; Instructor
in Psychology, Department of Psychiatry, Harvard Medical School,
Boston, Massachusetts

Robert J. Gregory, M.D.
Professor of Psychiatry, Upstate Medical University, Syracuse, New York

Rocco Iannucci, M.D.
Director, Fernside Addiction Recovery Program, McLean Hospital,
McLean Hospital, Belmont, Massachusetts; Instructor in Psychiatry,
Harvard Medical School, Boston, Massachusetts

Julia Jurist, B.A.
Clinical Research Assistant, Gunderson Personality Disorders Institute,
McLean Hospital, Belmont, Massachusetts

Sam Mermin, B.A.
Business Office Manager, Gunderson Personality Disorders Institute,
McLean Hospital, Belmont, Massachusetts

Grace Murray, B.A.
Ph.D. Student in Clinical Psychology, Boston University, Boston,
Massachusetts

Edward Patzelt, Ph.D.
Clinical Psychologist, Private Practice, Chicago, Illinois

Daniel Price, M.D.
Assistant Professor, Tufts University School of Medicine, Portland,
Maine; Psychiatry Residency Training Director, Maine Medical Center,
Portland, Maine

Kimberly Siscoe, M.D.
Psychiatrist, LifeStance Health, San Francisco, California

Georgia Steigerwald
B.A. Student, Harvard University, Cambridge, Massachusetts

Erik Ydrefelt, M.Sc. Psych
Clinical Psychologist, MBT Program, Outpatient Clinic for Emotional Instability, Malmö, Sweden; Team Director, National Program for Specialist Care of Severe Self-Injury, Lund, Sweden

Disclosures

The following contributors have indicated a financial interest in or other affiliation with a commercial supporter, manufacturer of a commercial product, and/or provider of a commercial service as listed below:

Lois W. Choi-Kain, M.D., M.Ed.
Consulting fees from Boehringer Ingelheim

Hilary S. Connery, M.D., Ph.D.
Funding from the National Institute on Drug Abuse; royalties from Guilford Press; consultant fees from Alosa Health

Jeffrey DeVido, M.D., M.T.S.
Stock or other financial options from Merck and Philip Morris/Altria

Carl Fleisher, M.D.
Employment with Reflect, Inc.

The following contributors stated that they had no competing interests during the year preceding manuscript submission:

Marcelo J. A. A. Brañas, M.D.; Stephen Conway, M.D.; Marcos S. Croci, M.D.; Robin Gay, Ph.D.; Robert J. Gregory, M.D.; Rocco Iannucci, M.D.; Julia Jurist, B.A.; Sam Mermin, B.A.; Grace Murray, B.A.; Edward Patzelt, Ph.D.; Daniel Price, M.D.; Kimberley Siscoe, M.D.; Georgia Steigerwald, B.A.; and Erik Ydrefelt, M.Sc. Psych

Preface

Borderline personality disorder (BPD) and alcohol use disorder
(AUD) co-occur quite often. Nearly half (46.4%) of all patients meeting
diagnostic criteria for BPD have a concurrent AUD, and more than half
(59.5%) will have AUD sometime in their life (Trull et al. 2018). The lifetime prevalence of alcohol dependence is estimated at 47% of people
with BPD (Trull et al. 2010). This rate makes alcohol dependence approximately five times more likely in those with BPD than in those without.
Among individuals with AUD or alcohol dependence, the prevalence of
BPD is nearly fivefold that of its prevalence in the community (Trull et al.
2018). Yet no integrated treatments for this common set of conditions—
which are practically the norm rather than the exception—have been adequately tested or disseminated.

BPD is prevalent, disabling, and sometimes fatal, but often treatable.
Six percent of North Americans will develop BPD in their lifetime (Grant
et al. 2008; Trull et al. 2010)—having BPD is a more common human
variation than blond hair. Fortunately, while still among the most stigmatized disorders in psychiatry and medicine at large, BPD has gained legit-
imacy as an important diagnosis through nearly four decades of scientific
study and treatment development. The prognosis for the disorder has
been radically transformed; despite the longstanding belief that it was
not treatable, we now know that it is highly likely to remit over time and
is responsive to numerous evidence-based psychotherapies. Nonetheless, BPD remains a disabling and sometimes fatal illness that shortens
life spans and opportunities. One in 10 people with BPD dies by suicide,
a risk exponentially greater than that of the general population. BPD remains a significant risk factor not only for self-destructive acts and death,
but also for other psychiatric and medical illnesses, violent crime and
victimization, and disability (Tate et al. 2022; Yen et al. 2021). The good
news is that those with BPD actively seek care in all settings, whether

psychiatric or medical. Therefore, health care professionals need a basic approach for providing sound treatment.

Alcohol use is a fixture in everyday life. Most adolescents and adults have access to alcohol, which is overused to a great extent (SAMHSA 2021). Binge drinking is common, with nearly half of those who use any alcohol meeting criteria for this pattern of overuse. Every health professional knows that alcohol use escalates the risk for numerous medical conditions; commonly co-occurs with other mood, anxiety, and substance use disorders; and contributes to destructive acts of aggression, violence, and suicide in addition to accidental injury (Rehm et al. 2014; World Health Organization 2014). Alcohol is the fourth leading cause of death (Pilar et al. 2020), which is largely preventable, since effective treatments exist to treat AUD. Alcohol use combines with the vulnerabilities of BPD bidirectionally to compound disabling symptoms, increase risk for death by suicide, and render treatment more challenging. But, like BPD, AUD is treatable. Numerous psychosocial and pharmacologic treatments have proven highly effective (see Kranzler 2023 for review). These treatments are vastly more available than those for BPD, and yet they are still grossly underutilized. Despite widespread recognition of AUD's detriments to physical and mental health, only one in five individuals with AUD ever receives treatment for the disorder (Grant et al. 2015).

These facts about BPD and AUD obviate the need for combined intervention. Both disorders are associated with significant stigma and misinformation. Called "the disorder doctors fear most" (Cloud 2009; Shanks et al. 2011), BPD is at the top of the medical conditions most stigmatized by health professionals themselves. To clinicians, those with BPD are often seen as "manipulative," but paradoxically, patients are sometimes "protected" from knowing their diagnosis because it is such bad news, despite the absence of any scientific evidence in favor of this practice. Research studies demonstrate that those who receive a BPD diagnosis are no less satisfied than those who receive other psychiatric diagnoses (Zimmerman et al. 2018). The devastating irony is that those with BPD will continue to have problems they cannot address or receive effective treatment for, and ultimately, they will suffer a self-image of being "broken beyond repair" and "unfixable" or hopeless instead (Gad et al. 2019).

Equally, AUD is considered through a screen of stigma. Those with AUD are more likely to be seen as responsible for their problems and not mentally ill, compared with individuals having other non–substance-related disorders (Kilian et al. 2021). Misinformation and stigma are the most common barriers to seeking treatment for those with AUD (Grant et al. 2015).

Myths about treating BPD and AUD, outlined in Table P–1, contribute to obstacles in seeking treatment for patients as well as active avoidance on the part of health professionals to provide combined intervention. These beliefs continue to influence care despite countervailing ideas backed by scientific investigations. Stigma, misinformation, and lack of training, combined with the usual challenges of treating these disorders, feed into the avoidance. Feelings of inadequacy and futility on the part of clinical professionals encountering individuals with these disorders contribute to significant unmet clinical needs for a subset of patients who, realistically, are likely to respond to treatment over time, if that treatment is tailored to incorporate help for both disorders. Medical illnesses commonly co-occur (e.g., diabetes and hypertension), and health care professionals know that the treatment of one without the other will severely limit the overall health benefits of intervention. The situation with BPD and AUD is no different: these are known psychiatric conditions with a vast scientific literature incorporated into national guidelines for treatment.

The *Handbook of Good Psychiatric Management for Borderline Personality Disorder and Alcohol Use Disorder*, has been written to overcome some of these obstacles by providing education and a general approach to the clinical management of patients with BPD and problematic alcohol use. It dispels common myths that discourage integrated BPD and AUD treatment (Table P–1) and provides rationales to encourage interventions using scientific evidence and national standards of care (Table P–2). The education we provide here is meant to be shared with patients, their loved ones, and clinical teams as a resource for motivation to persevere with the difficult but worthwhile investment in treatment.

This handbook is a starting point of care that can be adapted by most health professionals in most settings. It is not a lengthy, specialized approach reserved for experts. This generalist intervention is meant to be "good enough," in the spirit of pediatrician and psychoanalyst Donald Winnicott discussing normal developmental transformations (Winnicott 1953). Although intensive support may be required initially to medically and psychologically stabilize patients with BPD and AUD, so that they are in the best position to avail themselves of effective treatments, good psychiatric management (GPM) encourages clinicians to gradually foster tolerable challenges for patients in their lives outside of treatment so that they can develop a sense of capability to manage those challenges on their own.

Table P–1. **Myths about treatment of BPD and AUD**

Myth	Myth-Buster
Personality disorders are enduring, inflexible, and pervasive.	Some individuals experience symptoms as a single episode, and some with less severe symptoms move in and out of diagnosis (Videler et al. 2019).
Patients with BPD improve only if given extended, intensive expert treatment.	This is true of only a subsample. Generalist approaches for BPD have proven as effective as specialist approaches in several rigorous trials. Informed, structured, coherent interventions provided by those interested in working with individuals with BPD are shown to be effective across trials (Oud et al. 2018).
AUD should be treated first, and then BPD.	BPD escalates AUD symptoms and vice versa (Lazarus et al. 2017; Stepp et al. 2005). Many basic interventions, such as diagnostic disclosure and psychoeducation for both disorders, along with medication-assisted treatment for AUD, are easily integrated in generalist settings, no matter the length of stay.
BPD can be treated primarily without a focus on AUD.	AUD impairs neurocognition and the task of processing emotions and interpersonal experiences inherent to the therapeutic interventions known to work for BPD (Stavro et al. 2013).
Patients with BPD who drink responsibly do not need monitoring of their alcohol use.	Individuals with BPD are more likely to develop AUD over their lifetime, with new onset occurring in 13% of individuals with BPD (over 7 years) vs. 6% with other personality disorders (Walter et al. 2009).
Suicidality and self-harm in BPD should be treated before alcohol use.	Treatment of alcohol use problems in BPD is a critical step in reducing risk for suicide, as any substance use is a known transdiagnostic risk factor for suicide (Borges et al. 2000; 2017; Isaacs et al. 2022).

Note.   AUD=alcohol use disorder; BPD=borderline personality disorder.
Source.   Adapted from Gunderson and Links 2014.

We advise against attempting to control or take over the well-being of patients with BPD and AUD. Their complex vulnerabilities and high-risk tendencies may make this tempting, but as patients encounter expectable frustrations, missteps, and setbacks, we advise professionals to be realistic, balancing attentiveness with allowances of independence. We also frame GPM as a roadmap incorporating clinical wisdom with scientific research, but we expect professionals to diverge and necessarily adjust lessons according to their needs with each patient. Explicitly,

Table P–2.   Top 10 reasons supporting combined intervention for BPD and AUD

Reason to intervene	Intervention
BPD and AUD commonly co-occur: 46% of people with BPD meet criteria for AUD, and 17% of people with AUD meet criteria for BPD (Trull et al. 2018).	Treat both disorders simultaneously. Combining their treatments is possible and optimal. GPM's multimodal approach naturally incorporates medication, individual therapies, clinical case management, family work, and mutual help groups.
BPD and AUD share common risk factors, including impulsivity, negative affectivity, and sensation seeking.	Intervene early with psychoeducation about the interaction between disorders as well as the unique vulnerabilities of those with BPD to the reinforcing and impairing effects of alcohol.
BPD worsens the severity and course of AUD, AUD worsens the severity and course of BPD, and circular effects between BPD and AUD increase negative outcomes for both (Lazarus et al. 2017; Stepp et al. 2005; Walter et al. 2009).	As a routine part of good care for those with BPD, check in regularly about alcohol use. Routinely screen for BPD in those with AUD in substance use disorder treatment settings. (See Appendix E for screening instruments.)
Alcohol elevates risk for suicide across psychiatric disorders (Borges et al. 2000; Edwards et al. 2020; Sinclair and O'Neill 2020), and BPD patients are at high risk for suicide.	Treatment of alcohol use problems in those with BPD is an intervention to reduce risk for suicide.
A positive association exists between alcohol use and NSSI, and this relationship is stronger when alcohol use problems are more severe (Bresin and Mekawi 2022).	Treatment of alcohol use problems in those with BPD is an intervention to reduce NSSI.
BPD and AUD share core features of diminished neurocognitive and emotional processing capacity and insufficient agency, self-esteem, and coherent sense of self (Schulze et al. 2016).	Consider alcohol use a potential factor limiting the effectiveness of psychotherapies for BPD. Alcohol use interferes with the process of psychotherapy for BPD.

Table P-2.   Top 10 reasons supporting combined intervention for BPD and AUD (*continued*)

Reason to intervene	Intervention
Both BPD and AUD are associated with diminished social networks (Beeney et al. 2018; Lazarus et al. 2016; Mowbray et al. 2014; Stout et al. 2012; Zywiak et al. 2002).	Multimodal treatment broadens the social networks of those with BPD and AUD (multiple clinical professionals providing care alongside loved ones) to reduce risk factors for relapse, increase support, and enhance recovery from both disorders.
Comorbid BPD and AUD is associated with a specific set of drinking motives, including coping and conformity (Kaufman et al. 2020).	Emphasize the development of different coping responses and more effective prosocial behaviors that are more likely to generate the interpersonal responses needed for individuals with BPD and AUD to build health in their sense of self and relationships.
As opposed to AUD without BPD, comorbid AUD and BPD is associated with increased alcohol-related problems, independent of frequency or quantity or drinking (Kaufman et al. 2020).	Focus on what happens when the patient drinks, not just how much they drink.
Patients with comorbid BPD and AUD differ in their level of identification with each diagnosis and the symptoms they have the most motivation to change.	Use motivational interviewing that focuses on drinking behaviors as well as self-destructive behaviors related to BPD. Together, examine the reasons for these behaviors and their effects on goals, sense of self, and relationships; this will generate both commitment and agency in the patient's treatment.

Note.   AUD = alcohol use disorder; BPD = borderline personality disorder; GPM = good psychiatric management; NSSI = nonsuicidal self-injury.

GPM is designed to be practical and predictable but, like anything else, is not foolproof or perfect. No treatment for any serious health condition is. We hope it will be good enough to improve the status of care for those with BPD and AUD using tools already established, available, and widely employed by the good clinical professionals providing care for patients who seek it.

Acknowledgments

It takes a team to make a vision a reality. Both of us have spent our careers so far integrating our training in understanding and treating personality disorders and substance use disorders. With recurrent challenges and more limited improvements than treating either illness separately, we don't think the status quo is good enough. We enlisted the help of many dedicated and expert clinicians working in diverse real-world settings across the globe to contribute to this effort to close the chasm between the tools we already use and the need and demand for more integrated care for borderline personality disorder (BPD) and alcohol use disorder (AUD), a combination so prevalent that it can be considered the norm rather than the exception. Working together on this adaptation of good psychiatric management (GPM) has been meaningful and fun, which has made the process even more satisfying and important. From old friends (Rocco Iannucci) to new friends (Robert Gregory) to a cherished team of trainers in GPM, as well as students-now-colleagues (Steve Conway and Edward Paltzelt), we thank you from the bottom of our hearts (and our laptops at the crack of dawn and weekends).

From LCK: I thank the Osborn family, who has been a source of inspiration in their coping and learning from the extremes of human vulnerability and fallibility on one end, and remarkable love, forgiveness, faith, loyalty, and survival on the other. Seeing their persistent efforts to stay connected to Anne (and her to them) was one of the most painful and moving experiences of my life. Anne's explorations of life's possibilities seemed to know few limits. Containing her vibrant instability was like trying to catch lightning. Even through the most difficult clinical moments, full of risk-taking, going beyond the rails, and conflicts when trying to stop her, I still felt a deep personal connection to Anne and her humanity. Despite all this, and maybe because of it, I got to see her as a person beyond her BPD diagnosis. She was so full of life, she would jump off any cliff with her snowboarding wizardry that only continued more broadly in life, even when she retired from her career as an athlete, taking huge risks without the snowboard or slopes. I suppose she was highly imprinted with a tendency to live on the edge. But with each setback and disappointment, when she flew too close to that edge, I felt her shine become more thin, dull, and exhausted, especially when she later developed AUD. Watching her slip away is a trauma that will stay with me forever. The bond with her family, though, to get through the trauma eventually transformed my experience of attachment to Anne Osborn into survival, recovery, and growth. Lesley and David are a major wind beneath my wings in all I do. They have converted the painful intensity of loving and losing Anne into a story of faith, fueling work to promote mental health services and supports. I will be forever grateful for their support of me, my work, and this project. This handbook would never be possible without their commitment to honoring Anne's memory and struggles through a philanthropic gift to fuel its development. Plus, David taught me to hold a golf club without the need for a death grip (it's a bird, apparently).

I also thank my family and close friends for sticking with me throughout the chaotic life I have lived chasing solutions and interventions to keep up running alongside my patients, developing the Gunderson Residence, an intensive clinical program that literally never closed and now rigorously cranks out academic work, while traveling the world with a message of hope and change for BPD and other personality disorders. Mike Kain, thank you for your patient and reliable companionship in life, one where we are dedicated to the work of academic medicine, spending many nights and weekends working, always together in promoting each other's earnest but sometimes aggravating efforts to push our patients and the community toward better physical and mental health and functional mobility despite the many serious adversities they face. Emma and Abbie, you have had to give up much time with us for our *work before love* affliction, but I am so very proud of the people you have become, with personalities that are full of beautiful honesty, confidence, humor, and some really great dance moves. And always and forever, I thank my mentor, former taskmaster, father figure, and dear friend John Gunderson for seeing in me something that made you push me as hard as possible to see how far I could grow. Holding my feet to the fire of this work, carrying your legacy, and working with colleagues to change the status of BPD and its care has been completely worth it. My only regret is that you are not here to see it.

From both of us: Our patients and their families have been a source of education and learning about the universally human vulnerabilities that contribute to risk for these disorders. Everyone will know someone with either BPD and AUD in their lifetime, and many will know some with both these struggles. Witnessing their earnest efforts, persistent challenges, and enormous suffering has catalyzed a motivation to build a clearer path for these patients, their families, and the many clinicians who want to help but don't have the practical tools to do so confidently. We hope this book makes you feel more confident that you can help and, in the process, see the person behind these serious, sometimes fatal, debilitating illnesses.

Lois W. Choi-Kain, M.D., M.Ed.
Hilary S. Connery, M.D., Ph.D.

Introduction to Good Psychiatric Management for Borderline Personality Disorder and Alcohol Use Disorder (GPM-AUD)

Lois W. Choi-Kain, M.D., M.Ed.
Hilary S. Connery, M.D., Ph.D.

Introduction

This book was inspired by failures related to our limitations as expert clinicians treating borderline personality disorder (BPD) and alcohol use disorder (AUD). Despite the best resources of well-staffed, dedicated teams of clinicians in one of the best psychiatric specialty hospital systems in the United States, we repeatedly encountered treatment nonresponse and fatality from people with co-occurring BPD and substance use disorders, particularly those with alcohol misuse. In the legacy of John Gunderson, who refused to accept that patients with BPD were untreatable but rather believed that our field needed to better understand and tailor treatments to their specific diagnosis, we worked together with a team of specialists, researchers, and clinicians in real-world clinical settings who shared our commitment to build better treatments to reduce deaths from BPD and AUD. We know that a systematic integrated clinical management approach, based on usual principles of good psychiatric management (GPM), can guide clinical professionals to provide care that serves as a "good enough" holding environment for patients and their families through the painful process of recovery and rehabilitation from these complex, but treatable, disorders.

We wrote this book because there is a dire need to treat borderline personality disorder and alcohol use disorder simultaneously. The co-occurrence of these two disorders is practically the norm rather than the exception, and clinicians need an informed synthesis of approaches. The absence of any well-tested approach to treating BPD and AUD simultaneously with available psychosocial and psychopharmacologic interventions that are known to be effective for these disorders is stunning, considering how commonly patients present with both disorders. Too often, patients with BPD are discharged from addiction treatments because of acuity of self-destructive or interpersonally reactive behavior, while patients in BPD specialist settings are turned away because of acuity of substance use issues. This leaves a chasm too wide for any patient to handle, let alone those prone to despair and feeling overwhelmed on their own. These patients deserve better, and we can do better.

This handbook simply integrates the standard of care for both disorders as a general approach to what we know is effective for most health care providers to offer patients in general clinical settings. We aim to offer instructions that are ready-made, reusing the packaged toolbox of good care for any psychiatric condition that most clinicians already know and use.

Most clinicians will recognize negative affectivity and impulsivity as psychological traits shared by those with both disorders. Within the substantial population of patients who use alcohol, those with BPD show higher levels of risk factors for developing alcohol use problems (Jahng et al. 2011; Stepp et al. 2005). Clinical experts and researchers have pointed to the relevance of these shared traits as etiologically central to the development of both disorders (Conrod and Nikolaou, 2016; Gunderson et al. 2018). Studies demonstrate that alcohol use in BPD amplifies affect dysregulation, producing higher variability of negative affect swings for individuals with BPD who use alcohol than for those who do not (Jahng et al. 2011). Even when controlling for negative affectivity and impulsivity, those with BPD have greater alcohol-related problems than those without BPD (Carpenter et al. 2017; Trull et al. 2018).

Interpersonal instabilities combine with affective dysregulation and impulsivity to create the perfect storm of risk factors for AUD. In the largest epidemiological study ever conducted on alcohol-related conditions, researchers found that a general personality disorder factor (which represents the distinctive interpersonal dysfunction that differentiates personality disorders from other psychiatric conditions) drives most of the association between substance dependence and personality disorders (Jahng et al. 2011). This is a significant finding that converges with the more recently replicated discovery that BPD represents this general factor of personality dysfunction and is distinctive as an entity that reflects both the core of self and interpersonal dysfunction and the severity index shared among all personality disorders (Sharp et al. 2015; Wright et al. 2016a). In addition, research has found that those with BPD (versus those without) are more likely to use alcohol to cope and to conform socially (Kaufman et al. 2020). These motives significantly explain the association between BPD and alcohol-related problems, even when controlling for impulsivity and emotional dysregulation (Kaufman et al. 2020). Some data even suggest that BPD may represent a distinct subtype of AUD (Morgenstern et al. 1997). These findings reinforce our clinical observations that self-regulatory difficulties combine with interpersonal hypersensitivities to make those with BPD powerfully vulnerable to significant problems with alcohol use.

The presence of BPD in a clinical profile escalates the likelihood of developing other psychiatric disorders. BPD's pattern of co-occurrence with other disorders is complex (Tate et al. 2022; Zanarini et al. 2004); a vicious cycle of interactions unfolds with the specific vulnerabilities BPD generates. Adolescents with BPD symptoms are more likely to develop alcohol-related problems than those without (Stepp et al. 2005). Alcohol use in adolescence then goes on to amplify BPD symptoms (Lazarus et al. 2017). In adulthood, those with BPD are more likely to develop AUD and be prone to greater frequency of drinking relapses than those with other personality disorders (Walter et al. 2009). In a study that evaluated the daily amount and rate of alcohol consumption in those with BPD versus those without, investigators found that participants with BPD reported a faster rate of alcohol consumption, which reflects a proneness to binge drinking and may be related to maximizing the generation of positive emotions while dampening negative ones (Carpenter et al. 2017).

Not only are those with BPD more vulnerable to the usually destabilizing effects of alcohol, but they also face detriments in functioning and treatment response that heighten the likelihood of chronicity, ongoing adversity, and lifelong disability. Those with BPD and AUD report more limited academic achievement and greater unemployment (Miller et al. 1993). Treatment effectiveness for BPD is highly affected by the presence of alcohol use—greater levels of treatment dropout and limited treatment response occur when BPD and AUD co-occur (Ryle and Golynkina 2000; Wnuk et al. 2013). Active and routine assessment of alcohol use in patients with BPD, and vice versa, is therefore essential during treatment to decrease symptoms, increase functioning, and optimize treatment retention and response.

Although some evidence-based psychotherapies for BPD have been adapted to treat addictions (see Appendix A), the number of randomized controlled trials (RCTs) for these adaptations have been small, inconclusive, and sometimes contradictory, and none has been replicated. The most visible of the BPD-specific psychotherapeutic interventions in North America is dialectical behavioral therapy (DBT) (Linehan 1993), with more published clinical trial outcomes data than any other manualized approach. Only one trial tested DBT specifically for BPD co-occurring with substance use disorder (SUD) (Linehan et al. 1999; Appendix Table A–2). DBT was superior to treatment as usual in reducing substance use according to both self-report and urinalysis, as well as in increasing social and global adjustment. However, the trial included only 12 patients in DBT, and its findings have not been replicated. The trial's authors developed an adaptation of DBT for SUDs (Dimeff and Linehan, 2008), but its publication with public access remains pending.

Other DBT trials include one that studied BPD patients with and without SUDs, finding no differences between DBT and treatment as usual in days with >5 drinks, alcohol problems, or drug problems in the month before the final assessment (van den Bosch et al. 2002). In a later trial, participants receiving DBT had better outcomes than those treated by experts in the community in terms of days abstinent from drugs or alcohol, proportion of days abstinent, and remission from SUDs (Harned et al. 2008). However, only 8 of the 101 participants met criteria for AUD, so the generalizability of this finding is unknown. These results do not justify the use of full-scale DBT for the treatment of co-occurring AUD and BPD over other more basic approaches.

Schema-focused therapy (Young et al. 2003), which has also been effective in the treatment of BPD (Giesen-Bloo et al. 2006), has been adapted to treat SUDs with BPD in a variant called dual-focus schema therapy (see Appendix Tables A–1 and A–4). Unfortunately, it was not superior to individual counseling in published trials (Ball et al. 2011).

The only treatment approach specifically developed and applied in a sample of patients with BPD and AUD is dynamic deconstructive psychotherapy (DDP; Gregory 2022; Appendix Table A–3). Developed by Robert Gregory, M.D., a contributor to the development of the approach in this book, DDP is a psychodynamic psychotherapy that incorporates an understanding of split object relations driving the symptoms of borderline personality problems with a biological perspective of how alcohol use interferes with neurocognition and emotional processing that is central to most psychotherapeutic intervention. DDP (see Chapter 3, "Integrating Dynamic Deconstructive Psychotherapy Into Good Psychiatric Management") was compared with treatment as usual in a small sample of 30 patients in terms of immediate treatment response over 12–18 months of active therapy, as well as in follow-up 18 months after the end of therapy. Gregory's DDP approach was superior to treatment as usual in reducing parasuicidal episodes, alcohol use, and health care utilization at the end of treatment. DDP was also superior to treatment as usual in reducing BPD symptom levels and heavy drinking behavior a year or more after treatment (Gregory et al. 2008; 2010). Although DDP presents emerging evidence of efficacy, it has not been widely disseminated.

Specialized approaches to treating BPD are considered the gold standard, but are not widely available (Iliakis et al. 2019). No specialist approach besides DDP has been adequately tested for the combination of BPD and AUD. Trials of DDP conducted outside the developer's institution are still needed to assess generalization of its effectiveness more widely. In the meantime, we know that generalist approaches perform comparably to these specialist manualized psychotherapeutic approaches (Choi-Kain et al. 2017; Oud et al. 2018). Ongoing avoidance of diagnostic disclosure of BPD and AUD when they co-occur is fueled by therapeutic nihilism, limited access to evidence-based treatment options, and the short-term nature of such options for patients who will predictably struggle with complex and ongoing vulnerabilities.

GPM's Empirical Base

GPM's existing evidence base is growing (Kramer 2024; Links and Ross 2024). *General psychiatric management* (also called *good psychiatric management*) (GPM) serves as a comparator intervention in the largest methodologically rigorous randomized controlled trial of DBT conducted outside Linehan's laboratory (McMain et al. 2009). Shelley McMain, the principal investigator, wanted to ensure that the trial distilled the effective ingredients of DBT, that is, skills training and behavioral shaping, as the driver of superiority rather than simply the effects of an informed, structured treatment delivered by clinicians who liked treating BPD patients. The GPM-informed structured generic approach was developed by Paul Links, M.D., based on the texts *Borderline Personality Disorder: A Clinical Guide* (Gunderson 2001), *Borderline Personality Disorder: A Clinical Guide, Second Edition* (Gunderson and Links 2008), and the American Psychiatric Association Practice Guideline (American Psychiatric Association 2023). GPM combines core principles from psychodynamic psychotherapy with an informed psychiatric case management approach to BPD, offered in a 1-hour, once-a-week outpatient appointment. DBT was conducted with a 5-hour treatment package (i.e., 2-hour group, 1-hour individual, 2 hours of phone coaching). These differences in format reflect not only significantly reduced intensity in GPM, but also greater generalizability to most clinical settings. The equivalence in outcome despite the difference in treatment intensity and dosing offers some evidence that effective treatment can work with less time, training, and specialization (see Appendix C for a link to the General Psychiatric Management Online Training Course).

The unexpected outcome of McMain's trial was that DBT and GPM yielded comparable improvements in self-harm, suicidality, BPD symptoms, symptom distress, depression, anger, and interpersonal functioning in addition to significant reductions in utilization of health care (e.g., emergency room visits and inpatient hospitalization) (McMain et al. 2009; 2012). These gains were sustained at 2 years after treatment and in some domains continued to improve, again with no differences between the two treatments (McMain et al. 2012). Remission, defined as meeting fewer than two criteria of BPD for at least a year, was achieved in almost two-thirds of patients in both treatments by the end of 3 years. The absence of statistically significant differences was jarring, but good news for the distribution of a generic or generalist care approach to BPD.

GPM was delivered as a year-long format in McMain's trial, and adherence to its manual was sustained (Kolla et al. 2009; Appendix B). Lower dropout rates were observed in GPM compared with DBT in patients with higher co-occurrence of Axis I disorders (Wnuk et al. 2013; Appendix Table A–5). This finding is significant, because those with BPD and AUD are more likely to drop out from effective treatments (Barnicot et al. 2011; Iliakis et al. 2021; Ryle and Golynkina 2000). In Lausanne, Switzerland, another research team developed an application of GPM in a 10-session variant (Kramer et al. 2011; 2017; 2021) that serves as a starting point of care in their specialized psychotherapy clinic for personality disorders. Using this approach, in a sample of 85 patients, Kramer et al. (2014) found significant changes in symptoms and interpersonal functioning with medium effect sizes. This improvement reflects a crucial remoralization effect at the start of treatment to motivate patients through the hard work of change. A brief psychoeducational and diagnostic step of care using GPM helps patients understand their problems, establish goals, and build an alliance with a clinician. Adherence to GPM principles, rated by the adherence scale developed for McMain's study (Kolla et al. 2009), explained 23% of the variance in reduction of BPD symptoms and 16% of the variance in general symptom improvement in their 10-session GPM format (Kolly et al. 2016).

The 10-session variant was also studied in a sample of 99 patients with BPD, 51 who met criteria for a co-occurring SUD and 48 who did not (Penzenstadler et al. 2018; Appendix Table A–5). Surprisingly, not only did the total sample of patients—both with and without an SUD—achieve comparable reductions in general symptoms, but those with BPD and SUDs also had a higher reduction in BPD symptoms and a greater improvement in therapeutic alliance. Effects on SUDs were not systematically measured. Although this preliminary study was conducted with a broader group of BPD patients with SUDs, it nonetheless reflects the promise of applying GPM to this significant segment of patients we all encounter with BPD and AUD. These findings, while needing replication, suggest that GPM for AUD and BPD is safe, feasible, and effective. The effects are likely to improve with our integration of basic standards of AUD care.

In John Gunderson's 2014 re-manualization of this approach (*Handbook of Good Psychiatric Management for Borderline Personality Disorder* [Gunderson and Links 2014]) for public dissemination after McMain's research was published, he revised the title from *general* to *good psychiatric management* in the spirit of promoting principles of sound care that helps clinicians think and make informed decisions in treating the individual needs of each patient. He was encouraged by the advent of manualized treatments for BPD, but he was dismayed to see clinicians pay more attention to the tactics and techniques than their own clinical judgment or the unique needs of the patient in the moment. Gunderson wanted GPM to be a principle-driven approach in which we assume clinicians can integrate what they know about the best practices in our field, the patient they are treating, and what works and is pragmatically sustainable in their clinical environment. The expectation is that with a sound, systematic framework, we all develop experienced wisdom that refines our work throughout our careers.

Learning GPM for BPD starts with an 8-hour course that is available at low cost online (see Appendix C for link to online course for GPM for adults). Our research shows that this course changes clinicians' attitudes and increases confidence in treating patients with BPD. Before and after the 8-hour course, hundreds of clinicians across different tertiary care and community hospital settings rated their attitudes and capabilities in working with patients who have BPD. After the GPM course, the clinicians' avoidance, dislike, and hopelessness regarding the care of patients with BPD diminished, and their feelings of competence, belief in their capacity to make positive differences, and belief that effective BPD treatments exist all improved (Keuroghlian et al. 2016). Clinicians earlier in their career showed greater improvements in feeling competent after the training than more seasoned clinicians. It may be that less experienced clinicians learn in GPM training what many more established colleagues learn through years of clinical experience.

In a different sample, we assessed the same attitudes 6 months after GPM training (Masland et al. 2018). Immediately after the 8-hour GPM training, clinicians again reported feeling more competent in treating patients with BPD, more willing to disclose the diagnosis of BPD, and more likely to believe effective treatments for BPD exist. Six months later, they reported increased willingness to disclose the diagnosis and take on new patients with BPD as well as decreased difficulty with empathy and discomfort in treating patients with BPD. Patients with BPD are hypersensitive to others' attitudes toward them, and evidence shows they can detect negative emotions in facial expressions more effectively and sensitively than those without BPD (Fertuck et al. 2013; Lynch et al. 2006). Changes in clinician attitudes likely influence the therapeutic alliance by helping clinicians feel more comfortable, prepared, and optimistic about BPD treatment.

The guidance provided here is presented with the intention to be flexible. Length of treatment and frequency of visits should be adapted for the sustainable parameters of each clinical setting. GPM's use is encouraged if it is effective in helping patients reduce symptoms, facilitating BPD's natural course. Like other medical interventions, other options should be considered if it is not reducing symptoms or achieving clinical goals. In this handbook, we provide a roadmap of basic interventions, including diagnostic disclosure, psychoeducation, management of self-destructive tendencies, multimodal treatment, and family involvement

Table 1–1.   Distinctive characteristics of GPM

Element	Distinctive Features
Case management	Focus is on the patient's life outside therapy, not primarily on the patient's psychology as in psychotherapies.
Psychoeducation	Patients and families are informed of BPD's genetic disposition, expected changes, and the relative merits of different approaches.
Goals	Symptom reduction and self-control are secondary goals required to attain the primary goals of success in work and partnerships.
Multimodality	Psychopharmacological practices are integrated as adjunctive alongside endorsements for group therapies and family coaching.
Duration and intensity	No specific length and intensity are prescribed; patient and therapist collaborate in judging whether a therapy is effective.
Interpersonal hypersensitivity	An explicit and consistent effort is made to connect the patient's emotions and behaviors to interpersonal stressors.

Note.   BPD = borderline personality disorder.
Source.   Gunderson and Links 2014. Used with permission.

(see Table 1–1). Distinctively, we also incorporate an evidence-based approach to use of medications for alcohol use disorder and binge-drinking (MAUD) with the usual conservative psychopharmacologic procedures used in GPM more generally.

In the original trial, genPM prioritized focus on self-destructive behaviors and emotional processing. This handbook, like the original, prioritizes more broadly the joint effort to increase awareness and understanding of feeling states related to self-destructive tendencies, but also connects those feeling states to sources of interpersonal stress and instability. Current practice of GPM also places greater emphasis on functional concerns than the original trial. In McMain's trial, the majority of patients broadly experienced significant symptom reduction and BPD remission; however, they still reported high levels of disability and functional impairment despite these improvements (McMain et al. 2012). In response to this finding, our current courses and this GPM handbook direct clinicians to attend to functional progress. The most important intervention clinicians and patients can work on to promote personality development is *getting a life*—that is, as even Freud knew, stable work to fuel a sense of competence and contribution, along with love. Gunderson adjusted this mantra ("love and work," Freud as quoted in Erikson 1950) to *work before love*, as the dilemma for those with BPD is that it is difficult to be a steady partner in a relationship without independent activities, interests, and ability to care for oneself.

GPM emphasizes that most professionals need to provide *good enough* care to most patients with BPD encountered in most clinical settings. Gunderson wrote in the original Handbook, "You don't need to be a specialist, to be selflessly devoted, or have a larger-than-life personality to be 'good enough'; you need to be warm, reliable, interested, and unintimidated" (Gunderson and Links 2014, p. 4). In developing this adaptation of GPM to provide early intervention for BPD with AUD, we hoped it would provide clarity in the face of challenge and confusion, and that it would steady clinicians in the face of expectable and usual challenges inherent in the treatment of BPD and AUD. GPM presents a means of socializing clinicians, patients, and their families to medicalized roles aimed expressly to improve health. Not only does medicalization provide clear roles and goals in the face of the interpersonal instability inherent in BPD, GPM's medicalized framework also destigmatizes the problems associated with both BPD and AUD as biologically based and environmentally shaped to reduce blame and empower patients to manage their symptoms.

For clinicians who are experienced with treating SUDs, GPM also offers a boiled-down introduction to managing BPD. GPM can be adapted in short-term acute settings such as emergency departments (Hong 2016; 2019) and inpatient units (Choi-Kain and Gunderson 2019), where usual evidence-based approaches to BPD cannot be applied. GPM can also be the basis of care in longer-term outpatient psychiatric clinics (Price 2019) and primary care settings (Adler et al. 2019). GPM maintains a flexible framework, to accommodate any clinical setting, duration, and intensity of care. With a practical care management approach that incorporates generic psychotherapeutic concepts and common factors found within most effective approaches across diagnoses, GPM focuses on helping clinicians and patients 1) promote motivation that treatment can work, 2) build a therapeutic alliance, 3) improve awareness of sources and mechanisms behind patients' difficulties, 4) reinforce consistent reality testing, and 5) broker corrective experiences that dispel mistrust of oneself and others (Goldfried 2019). Although GPM incorporates these basic psychotherapeutic common factors, it need not be thought of as an individual therapy, but rather as just good standard clinical care. This adaptation for AUD also incorporates basic principles derived from DDP, the only BPD-focused, evidence-based approach tested with positive results (Appendix Table A–2; see Chapter 3, "Integrating Dynamic Deconstructive Psychotherapy Into Good Psychiatric Management").

Central to understanding GPM is the idea that those with BPD are born with innate, partially neurobiological dispositions that make them sensitive to situational stressors, particularly to problems in relationships (e.g., family environment and school). An individual's stress sensitivity also makes them vulnerable to developing AUD if exposed to the powerful reinforcing effects of alcohol and its widespread availability. These dual sources of sensitivity feed patients' insecurity in relationships and in their growing sense of self, in ways that destabilize their navigation toward a stable and rewarding life.

Importantly, GPM employs skepticism about any inclination to become dependent on treatment or form an identity primarily as a patient. This happens frequently when patients go from one failed or only temporarily effective treatment to another. Instead, it encourages clinicians to minimize harm first and emphasizes how surprisingly helpful treatment can be by avoiding common clinical maneuvers such as unguided polypharmacy, repeated hospitalization, and care that is not tailored to these two key destabilizing psychiatric disorders, and instead to disorders (such as depression) that are unlikely to remit without treatment of BPD or AUD.

GPM-AUD's Place in Treatment Planning

GPM-AUD is not an ambitious treatment approach. It strives to be generic and entry level, accessible to all patients and all health professionals. GPM is not meant to be the best treatment ever constructed for these disorders, but rather one that is good enough for most clinicians to learn and use, most patients to access and receive, and most health care settings to pragmatically incorporate as a standard of treatment. In some settings, for some patients, those who fail should be referred to a higher level of care (see Chapter 9, "Level-of-Care Considerations for Patients With Substance Use Disorder and Borderline Personality Disorder").

Realistic expectation of being adequate, well-intentioned, and reasonably informed is what most patients should have for their health care providers. All patients need to understand that all treatments have limitations and flaws. No treatment works all the time, for all patients, at all points of their clinical trajectory. Those with BPD, who have a distinctive tendency to idealize and devalue others in important relationships, need to understand this as a road to recovery, so they can see that normal disagreement or disappointment does not represent persecution, abuse, neglect, or sinister motives. BPD's best-known treatments for adults are lengthy and psychotherapeutically elaborate, but research shows that intensity and duration does not determine outcome (Cristea et al. 2017). Evidence also shows that with intermittent, shorter-term, usual nonintensive treatments available in the community, those with BPD can improve (Bender et al. 2006; Paris 2013). Intensive treatment provides a holding zone to reassess, regroup, and plan a way forward but is not meant to be a haven that is always there when times get tough. As Gunderson noted in the original handbook (p. 4), GPM practitioners are provided this key mantra: "[L]ife's lessons can be a great ally to bring about change if they become integrated. Treaters facilitate learning these lessons."

GPM-AUD incorporates fundamental concepts of what works in DBT, mentalization-based treatment (MBT), and transference-focused psychotherapy (TFP) in an introductory education for clinicians, so that if needed and available, GPM-AUD as a first step of care can pave the way to further work with those treatment approaches. GPM-AUD also offers a means of ongoing, less-intensive follow-up after such treatments end, as they are finite. Most importantly, GPM can serve as primary care for health maintenance, symptom management, and triage as needed. GPM-AUD fulfills a pragmatic role, flexible enough to meet the situational demands of a patient's life at various stages of their recovery from both BPD and AUD but firm enough to contain the expectably tumultuous and challenging process. For clinicians, GPM-AUD presents the opportunity to work from a generalist framework over the course of a patient's life span, even when BPD's most salient features or alcohol use problems may remit but their core vulnerabilities of stress sensitivity remain.

BPD's criteria reflect the maladaptive self and interpersonal function generally characteristic or shared among all personality disorders (Sharp et al. 2015; Sharp and Wall 2018). GPM is therefore relevant for the treatment of all personality difficulties, since it focuses on general personality function of managing oneself (i.e., coping, self-direction, identity) as well as relations with others, or lack thereof (i.e., related to capacity for empathy and intimacy) irrespective of specific flavors determined by traits.

With a pragmatic direction, GPM is designed to support symptom management to pave a stable road for Freud's *love and work*, or in Gunderson's words, *getting a life*.

GPM's Foundations in Longitudinal Research

Gunderson's studies describing BPD's phenomenology and features, formalizing diagnostic assessments, charting its longitudinal course, differentiating BPD from commonly co-occurring disorders, and estimating its familiality and heritability provided the evolving scientific basis of his clinical management of patients with the disorder. Gunderson introduced the first versions of GPM's interpersonal hypersensitivity model, with descriptions of how BPD's symptoms fluctuated with relational shifts to important attachment figures, in his landmark clinical guide *Borderline Personality Disorder*, first published in 1984 to precede any other manualized treatment approach (Gunderson 1984). This core formulation is the foundation of GPM's longstanding approach as well as its many current adaptations (Choi-Kain and Gunderson 2019; Choi-Kain and Sharp 2021; Sonley and Choi-Kain 2021). This enduring framework is preserved in this book and integrated with an understanding of its interaction with alcohol use.

Longitudinal prospective follow-up studies of the naturalistic course of BPD in comparison with other personality disorders and co-occurring mood, anxiety, and behavioral conditions organize a broader clinical management approach. In the Collaborative Longitudinal Study of Personality (CLPS; Gunderson et al. 2000), Gunderson and colleagues demonstrated that those with BPD can experience enduring symptomatic remission in as little as 6 months without extended intensive evidence-based therapies, with sudden life changes and medication changes or other clinical interventions (Gunderson et al. 2003). In fact, most who met criteria for BPD at the start of these studies no longer met criteria after a decade's time, suggesting that the natural course of BPD was remission (Gunderson et al. 2011; Zanarini et al. 2012). BPD's most distinguishing features—that is, frantic efforts to avoid abandonment and unstable relationships characterized by idealization and devaluation, also known as its interpersonal features—are predictive of the level of BPD symptoms persisting after 2 years. Furthermore, the quality of relationships at baseline significantly predicted functioning 2 years later (Gunderson et al. 2006). Interpersonal factors contribute significantly to the maintenance of BPD symptoms over the long-term course. This finding affirms GPM's notion of interpersonal hypersensitivity as a central engine of BPD.

The major findings from CLPS on the interaction between BPD and its common co-occurring disorders underpins GPM's approach to organizing management of BPD's usually complex pattern of co-occurrence with other psychiatric conditions, of which AUD is among the most common. BPD symptoms predict persistence of depressive symptoms at follow-up, but not vice versa (Gunderson et al. 2004). This finding suggests that clinicians can treat BPD to facilitate remission from depression. Compared with patients without BPD, patients with BPD have greater rates of new onset of both alcohol and drug use disorders over time, as well as shorter time to develop them, whether remitted or not (Walter et al. 2009). Treating BPD and systematically evaluating alcohol and drug use even after remission is critical to achieving the greatest stabilization for this group of patients.

Importantly, functional recovery is far less common and stable than symptomatic remission in longitudinal studies (Gunderson et al. 2011; Zanarini et al. 2012); therefore, clinicians using GPM support and encourage patients to assume responsibilities outside treatment in ways that foster learning how to function through adaptation and maturation. Clinical experience teaches us that reduction of symptoms alone may not lead to increased functioning and is achieved in some cases by removing functional demands, adding sedating and cognitively impairing medications, and occupying patients chronically in intensive clinical programs that may continue to handicap patients with BPD inadvertently in the long run, as well as paradoxically interfere with the development of adaptive personality functioning.

GPM's Relationship to Treatment Guidelines and Other Evidence-Based Options for BPD

The updated American Psychiatric Association Practice Guideline for the Treatment of Patients with BPD (American Psychiatric Association 2023) reports limited evidence to support the use of medications as a primary treatment for BPD and advises using them in intervention for co-occurring disorders combined with the use of psychosocial intervention to target BPD. GPM-AUD is the only manualized approach to meet these recommendations for AUD co-occurring with BPD. The obvious advantage is that GPM uses care management as a more critical component than any medication or individual therapy. GPM-AUD parsimoniously advises targeted medication management for AUD according to guide-lines for its care (see Chapter 7, "Pharmacotherapy for Co-occurring Borderline Personality Disorder and Alcohol Use Disorder") and encour-ages the use of sobriety support groups (see Chapter 8, "Multimodal Treatments"). Psychotherapy on an individual basis, even when recom-mended, often remains inaccessible at preliminary steps of care even in the best health care systems in the world (Hermens et al. 2011).

Specialized psychotherapies such as DBT, MBT, and TFP will always be forerunners of the core innovations of BPD care that have driven prog-ress in its understanding and treatment. GPM borrows a highly selective set of tactics and techniques from these approaches (see Table 1–2). GPM emphasizes the need for patients to think first, to better understand how interactions with others influence symptomatic crises, and then to think through what can be done to be more effective in using prosocial rather than socially destructive and isolating behaviors. GPM's emphasis on in-terpersonal transactions overlaps significantly with both MBT's and TFP's attention to improving the coherence and realistic lens through which people with BPD can understand attachment and close relations. GPM centralizes the concept of splitting in its formulation, connecting the way patients with BPD experience relational interactions in idealized and devalued terms, stemming from anxious and angry emotional states. In contrast to MBT, GPM encourages clinicians to make interpretations but does so in terms of the patient's predictable symptomatic abandon-ment fears and intolerance of aloneness. Lastly, GPM instructs clinicians to manage boundaries and countertransference reactions by teaching them to anticipate urges to protect or rescue as well as reject or punish based on these splits.

GPM uses a not-knowing stance, encouraging clinicians to express their views as a fallible subjective perspective rather than an authorita-tive truth. Common to all the approaches is validation of the patient's point of view, while also promoting the tolerance of the clinician's sense of separateness in perspective. Healthy skepticism is always an antidote to idealizing tendencies and promotes independent reappraisal of situa-tions as well as normal disagreement in the service of teaching patients a more realistic and sustainable way of managing their relationships with others. Importantly, GPM and these other treatments foster effective and relationally thoughtful moves in the service of self-assertion. Realis-tic estimation of the attribution of motives and intentions behind one's own and other's actions, delivered in candid direct conversation using an attitude of interest and curiosity, is the hallmark of GPM, which cuts out

Table 1-2.   GPM's integration of prior evidence-based psychotherapies

Modality	Concept	Therapeutic stance	Interventions
TFP	Splitting and projection as defenses against anger	Monitoring boundaries and countertransference	Interpretation of anger; challenge avoidance and acting out
DBT	Social and psychological skill deficits	Coaching	Self-monitoring; homework; intersession availability
MBT	Theory of mind; attachment	Not knowing	Examining attributions about self and others

Note.   DBT = dialectical behavioral therapy; GPM = good psychiatric management for borderline personality disorder; MBT = mentalization-based treatment; TFP = transference-focused psychotherapy.

Source.   Adapted from Gunderson and Links 2014.

more complex psychotherapeutic techniques embodied in the specialized therapies.

Ultimately, GPM embraces the notion that individuals with BPD and AUD may have arrested development of critical social and psychological skills that can be reactivated through social learning. As noted earlier, GPM widely embraces what works and makes sense from other treatments with a less-is-more attitude that embraces the medical guideline of minimal optimal dosing. GPM's pragmatism and eclecticism foster the ability to combine available clinical resources with selected tools from specialist therapies that can be scaled in intensity as needed (see Chapter 9, "Level-of-Care Considerations for Patients With Substance Use Disorders and Borderline Personality Disorder").

No RCT has yet studied this adaptation of GPM for BPD and AUD. We hope there will be such a study to justify its use in the future. We hope that this book may enable empirical research using GPM-AUD. For now, we aim to use current community standard-of-care approaches to provide an integrated-care framework for treatment of BPD+AUD that serves to close the treatment gap and guide future clinical research. GPM's equivalence to DBT in outcomes in adults with a variety of usual co-occurring illnesses suggests its suitability for use but needs to be enhanced by standard-of-care interventions for AUD, including both

Table 1–3. Key adjustments in adapting GPM to treat co-occurring BPD and AUD

1.	Attention to alcohol use regardless of meeting full criteria for AUD	Those with BPD are at a heightened risk for new-onset AUD (Walter et al. 2009) and may have a problematic relationship with alcohol that interferes with psychotherapy even if it does not meet criteria for AUD.
2.	Translation of materials into relatable language	Keeping the concepts focused and simple enables patients and clinicians to invest in a few points repeatedly rather than many points superficially.
3.	Involvement of the social network	Expanding the patient's social network of others who will support their recovery may stabilize the oscillations of BPD symptoms and the drivers of alcohol use.
4.	Active incorporation of MAUD	The standard of care for AUD management includes the use of pharmacology (outlined in Chapter 7). These medications can be prescribed by primary care physicians or others on a regular basis in conjunction with any psychosocial treatment.
5.	Explicit focus on life outside of treatment in a manner that builds a sense of self and a vision of the future	This effort will bolster the patient's reasons not to drink or not to engage in self-destructive or self-defeating behavior. Trying to isolate or insulate the patient from life's stressors may only keep the patient vulnerable to feeling lost and purposeless when facing high urges to relapse.

Note. AUD = alcohol use disorder; BPD = borderline personality disorder; GPM = good psychiatric management for BPD; GPM-AUD = good psychiatric management for BPD + AUD; MAUD = medication for AUD.

MAUD and psychosocial interventions as available (Table 1–3). We hope that in this moment, it provides a confidence-building approach for clinicians who want to follow guidelines for treating patients with this challenging combination of conditions, and to do so in a way that is accessible, pragmatic, and effective.

We hope that this handbook provides you with the wisdom you need to feel confident and competent, with an up-to-date fund of knowledge and a clear framework for understanding both BPD and AUD. This knowledge is the foundation you can use to psychoeducate patients and their families about the biological disposition at the root of their vulnerabilities, which they can learn to manage like any other medical condition to enhance neurocognitive, psychological, and personality functioning in a way that optimizes mental health, self-worth, and supportive and durable social bonds. Although both disorders will potentiate risk for treatment nonresponsiveness, disability, morbidity, and mortality, implementation of the best practices for treating BPD and AUD simultaneously will enable most clinicians to offer good-enough treatment that is most likely to engage and stabilize this difficult population.

Finally, recognizing that self-injury and suicide risk are elevated in BPD and AUD populations, we also provide the reader with clear, evidence-based approaches to suicide prevention and clinician strategies to mitigate liability risk, the necessary knowledge all clinicians require to confidently work with patients having life-threatening illnesses. We believe that with these tools, most clinicians are good enough to do effective work with patients with BPD and AUD, who may otherwise remain disabled, demoralized, and at risk for premature death. This is the aim of most mental health professionals, who are simply in need of coherent guidelines and tools informed by research. As John Gunderson would have said, we hope you find this useful.

2

Overall Principles

Marcelo J. A. A. Brañas, M.D.
Kimberley Siscoe, M.D.
Erik Ydrefelt, M.Sc. Psych
Marcos S. Croci, M.D.
Lois W. Choi-Kain, M.D., M.Ed.

Good Psychiatric Management Theory: Interpersonal Hypersensitivity

The oscillations of the diverse affective, interpersonal, behavioral, and cognitive/self-dysfunctions of borderline personality disorder (BPD) confuse, irritate, and scare clinicians who will benefit from making sense of patients' seemingly unpredictable episodes of emotional turmoil. When alcohol use disorder (AUD) co-occurs with BPD, clinical decompensations can be even more severe and life-threatening. Having a model to understand the complex nature of BPD's symptoms and its changeability helps clinicians be more grounded in the usual principles of good psychiatric care they already use for other conditions.

BPD develops out of a transaction between biological vulnerability and adverse or unsupportive social processes. Its heritability rates are moderately strong, with studies showing a range from 0.42 to 0.69 (Distel et al. 2008; Kendler et al. 2011; Skoglund et al. 2021; Torgersen et al. 2000). Interpersonal symptoms are those that best discriminate the disorder from other diagnoses (Zanarini et al. 1990). Factors such as insecure attach-

19

ment, childhood adversity, negative experiences, and familial dysfunction are predictive of the diagnosis (Agrawal et al. 2004). Neurobiologically, patients with BPD have heightened sensitivity to perceived threats in interpersonal situations (Daros et al. 2013), related to negative bias in interpreting interpersonal cues, enhanced amygdala responses, and poor regulation of limbic areas by the prefrontal cortex (Bertsch et al. 2013).

Having BPD causes individuals to be more pervasively vulnerable to multiple psychiatric conditions and to have more chronicity in their illness trajectory. New onset of AUD and substance use disorders (SUDs) in patients with BPD is higher than in those with other personality disorders (Walter et al. 2009). SUDs and BPD share deficits in social processing, that is, the ability to recognize, interpret, and convey appropriate social information (Hanegraaf et al. 2021). In both disorders, the capacity to understand one's own emotions and intentions is impaired, leading to worse social outcomes (Pennay et al. 2011).

The interpersonal hypersensitivity (IHS) model (Gunderson 2007; Gunderson and Lyons-Ruth 2008) is the theoretical framework of good psychiatric management for BPD (GPM-BPD, or in this book, simply GPM). The IHS model endeavors to integrate the vacillating clinical phenomena frequently encountered in individuals with BPD; it may also provide a helpful framework for treating individuals with SUDs complicating BPD. What empirically validated treatments for BPD have in common is a coherent formulation of the symptoms BPD patients face, allowing clinicians and patients to organize therapeutic interventions around a shared framework, to understand self-harming and emotional crises, to provide accurate psychoeducation, and to promote effective, collaborative patient-clinician interactions (Gunderson and Links 2014).

Interpersonal Hypersensitivity Model and the Development of Borderline Personality Disorder

The IHS model explains the complex nature of BPD as organized around a core mechanism of interpersonal vulnerability. This understanding of BPD emerged from Gunderson's early observation of the changeability of patients' presentation according to interpersonal contexts (Gunderson 1984).

Modern understanding of personality development involves two domains: interpersonal relatedness and self-definition. This perspective is reflected in alternative proposals in diagnostic manuals (i.e., DSM 5-TR, Section III [American Psychiatric Association 2022] and ICD-11 [World Health Organization 2022]), which focus on self and interpersonal functioning as the core of personality pathology (Sharp 2022). In both BPD and SUDs, patients have a diminished capacity for self-knowledge, albeit via different neural mechanisms (Hanegraaf et al. 2021). Having self-clarity is vital for effective social interactions (de Guzman et al. 2016). Interpersonal relationships are the context in which a robust self can develop (Luyten and Blatt 2013). Functioning on an individual level and functioning on an interpersonal level bidirectionally influence each other in both positive and negative ways.

In BPD, interpersonal hypersensitivity makes the patient prone to relational stressors, which can lead to different stages of symptomatic decompensation (see Figure 2–1).

Initially, the patient may present in a socially cooperative and anxiously attached *connected* state. They may exhibit compliance, neediness, and a version of themselves that reflects some mastery and stable self-esteem (Table 2–1). However, rejection sensitivity fosters hypervigilance and anxiety about threats to important and valued relationships. Real or perceived rejection or criticism, loneliness, ambiguity, and lack of structure can threaten this connectedness, leading to sudden shifts in interpersonal behavior. Anger that arises in the face of threats is turned inward, with states of self-harming, desperation, and disintegration, or turned outward to others in argumentative, blaming, and devaluing behavior.

Next in the model is a fight-or-flight stress-reactive state for a patient with BPD. In this *threatened* state, neurocognitive function (involved in both top-down regulation and executive function) is impaired, leading them to have significant difficulties in realistically appraising the situation at hand (Table 2–1). With faulty and emotionally reactive interpretations of events, they are prone to adopting maladaptive or destructive coping methods, such as substance misuse. Alcohol intoxication further impairs capacity for realistic self-appraisal with regard to motivation, judgment, and accurate interpretation of other people's intentions or behaviors.

People in the patient's social orbit, including clinicians, find these stress-reactive fight-or-flight behaviors challenging to tolerate, because they naturally elicit anxious, angry, or fearful reactions. If others express concern by leaning in to understand and work through the problems at hand, a patient may return to a *connected* state. However, often, others will withdraw from or reject the patient, who will then descend into a state of *aloneness*. Those with BPD distinctively cannot tolerate aloneness because of an undeveloped sense of self and incapacity to feel secure without others (Gunderson 1996). This alone state, in which the patient is unanchored from the realistic consequences of their actions and is un-

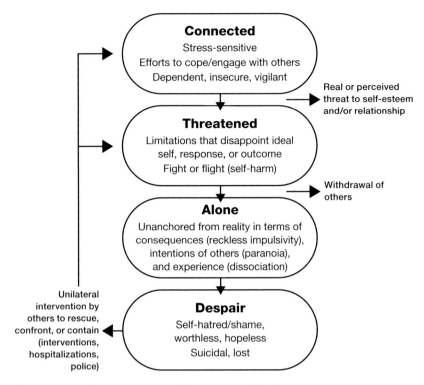

Figure 2–1.   **Interpersonal hypersensitivity model for BPD + AUD.**

Note.   AUD = alcohol use disorder; BPD = borderline personality disorder.
Source.   Adapted from Gunderson and Links 2014.

able to estimate what is going on for others, results in paranoia, dissociation, and reckless impulsivity, which may include alcohol use. Alcohol intoxication frequently amplifies feelings of despair, hopelessness, and lacking reasons to live. This despair state carries more dangerous suicidal risk than the threatened state, when the patient is still engaged and actively working toward a solution to the problem generating their stress reaction.

All too often, clinical interventions occur when the patient is already acting in a recklessly impulsive way. In states of *aloneness* or *despair*, others generally need to take control and enact unilateral action to rescue or contain the patient with BPD+AUD. The holding effect and show of care of such measures lead the patient to feel more valued and worthwhile; thus they are relieved of aloneness, which is difficult for them to tolerate without maladaptive coping. The stabilizing effects of these interventions may return the patient to a workable state in the short run, but in

Table 2–1. States of BPD+AUD's interpersonal hypersensitivity model

Interpersonal state	Definition	Implications for treatment
Connected	The patient feels "held" and contained by an idealized relationship. In this connected state, the patient is collaborative, dependent, and rejection sensitive.	Patient is relatively accessible; they need a social safety net and expanded treatment community.
Threatened	The patient encounters real or perceived hostility, rejection, or abandonment, resulting in aggressive behaviors toward others and themselves (e.g., anger, self-harm).	
Alone	If the patient's behavior elicits withdrawal, the patient becomes distressed, dissociated, and help-rejecting. At this stage, the patient is more difficult to reach or influence.	Unilateral action to contain or rescue may eliminate autonomy and agency.
Despair	Without a containing relationship, when truly alone, the patient becomes anhedonic and seriously suicidal.	

Note. AUD=alcohol use disorder; BPD=borderline personality disorder.
Source. Adapted from Choi-Kain and Gunderson 2019.

the long run can lead to a chronic dependence on others and clinical units as a recurrent external solution to internal problems. This dependence generates iatrogenic harms such as reinforcing self-identity as a disabled "patient" and limiting opportunities for autonomous functioning.

The Interpersonal Hypersensitivity Model and Alcohol Use Disorder

Individuals with BPD may initially use alcohol to alleviate social anxiety, cope with painful experiences, or conform to societal norms (Chugani et al. 2020; Kaufman et al. 2020). Alcohol use can lead to significant detriments to health, well-being, and psychosocial functioning, leaving patients with limited interpersonal connections and structure (Rehm 2011).

Because those with BPD crave and drink more rapidly than those without BPD, alcohol use may ignite more rapid oscillations into diminished neurocognitive processing, impulsivity, and detachment (Carpenter et al. 2017; Lane et al. 2016; Thompson et al. 2017; Wilson et al. 2006). Denial, reckless behavior, and shame impede the process of repair and reconnection and can result in frequent control struggles and repeated dropouts from treatment (Gregory 2019). GPM-AUD uses the enhanced IHS model to enable patients and clinicians to talk about the role and impact of alcohol use on the usual oscillations of stress-reactive states in both disorders. Table 2–2 describes potential functions that patients may seek when consuming alcohol and points out their impact in BPD psychopathology along the continuum of interpersonal states of connection and disconnection.

Alcohol use not only catalyzes the speed with which patients transition between these interpersonally hypersensitive states, it also impairs neurocognitive functioning such that patients are further challenged in processing their emotions, accurately reading internal and social cues, and developing effective responses to stressful situations. The progression of alcohol's effects varies from individual to individual. For some, alcohol may initially have rewarding effects to diminish negative emotions, enhance positive ones, and relieve social anxiety. As individuals with BPD use alcohol with these rewarding effects, however, the usual neurocognitive effects of intoxication result in a loss of control over use. In threatened states, the person with BPD using alcohol may become more impulsively aggressive or self-harming, and the escalation to more self-destructively impulsive, dissociative, and paranoid tendencies in the state of *aloneness* is fueled by alcohol even in the absence of rejection or withdrawal from others (Figure 2–2). Alcohol use may precipitate a state of unreachability earlier for those with BPD, so the true suicidal despair becomes more dangerous, and unilateral rescue or confrontation by others becomes necessary to keep the patient alive. For moderate to severe AUD, the initial states of rewarding effects may be absent, as dependence is what drives use rather than positive effects. As higher quantities of alcohol are needed to manage dependence, control over use is lost.

Both BPD and AUD involve dilemmas of control and ambivalence about autonomy. Because control is gained unstably through self-harm, aggression, and alcohol use in threatened states, individuals with both disorders will be further impaired in their ability to build a positive, stable sense of self, as well as meaningful and durable relationships with others. The enhanced interpersonal hypersensitivity model incorporates attention to the potentiating and interactive effects of alcohol use for those with BPD.

Table 2–2. Functions and consequences of alcohol use in BPD

Interpersonal state	Desired effects of alcohol	Consequences of alcohol use
Connected	To suppress general anxiety, loosen social inhibition, sensation-seeking, craving; increase a subjective sense of control	Increased interpersonal vulnerability, depression, superficial social connection
Threatened	To manage difficult feelings and thoughts, suppress attachment needs, socially conform, stop craving	Disinhibited anger toward self and others, NSSI, impulsive sexual activity, suicidal threats
Alone	To manage severe emotional pain (e.g., loneliness, emptiness, dissociation, paranoia)	Lack of control over drinking and coping in general and increased disconnection from others and reality
Despair	To self-destruct, not caring to live unless rescued	Lack of agency, disinhibition of suicidal acts, stuck in overwhelming pain

Note. BPD = borderline personality disorder; NSSI = nonsuicidal self-injury.

Basic Therapeutic Approach

GPM-AUD embodies eight basic principles that practitioners can use to guide the treatment of those with BPD and AUD (Table 2–3).

Offer Psychoeducation

Sharing the BPD+AUD diagnosis and your knowledge about its causes, course, and treatment with patients and families is a fundamental starting point of clinical intervention. Psychoeducation is a cost-effective preliminary step of treatment that effectively reduces BPD symptoms (Ridolfi et al. 2019; Zanarini et al. 2018; Zanarini and Frankenburg 2008). Informing patients about the disorder for which they are in treatment in a constructive, informed, and professional manner instills hope and establishes expectations to make the most out of the treatment.

Framing these conditions in a medical model reduces stigma and shame. When informed about prevalence, the role of genetics, and basic neurobiology (e.g., overactive amygdala underregulated by the prefron-

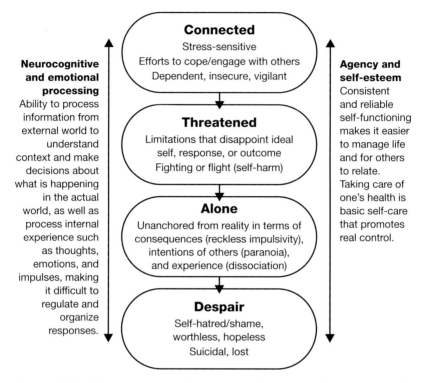

Figure 2–2. Processing and agency relevant to interpersonal hypersensitivity in BPD+AUD.

Note.   AUD=alcohol use disorder; BPD=borderline personality disorder.
Source.   Adapted from Gunderson and Links 2014.

tal cortex, reward circuitry), patients learn that others have the same problem and that their condition is not a "character flaw," which helps lessen guilt and saves them from the dichotomy of fatalistic thinking or masochistic self-blaming. Furthermore, by knowing how their illness works (e.g., interpersonal coherence model, embedded badness, neuro-cognitive deficits), patients can identify triggers and more readily soothe themselves using healthier alternatives (e.g., crises/safety plan) and pro-actively work on problem-solving.

GPM clinicians are encouraged to focus on functional rehabilitation (especially vocational) as a preliminary step to stabilizing relationships. Instead of adopting an authoritative and controlling stance, taking the role of a consultant to the patient fosters both autonomy and collaboration while not openly taking sides in the patient's ambivalence toward treatment. This is the essence of motivational interviewing.

Table 2-3. Basic principles of GPM-AUD

Principle	Comment
1. Offer psychoeducation	Don't hesitate to inform patients about what you know (or don't know) about their diagnoses and treatment. Give advice when you feel it will be instructive. Allow the patient to decide to agree or disagree.
2. Be active, not reactive	Being responsive assures patients that you are interested and involved; do not catastrophize.
3. Be thoughtful	You are a container for your patient's anxiety and a role model for "thinking first."
4. The relationship is real as well as professional	Both aspects—real and professional—are necessary.
5. Convey that change is expected	The absence of change raises questions about the treatment's value. Change will be gradual, and ambivalence is to be expected.
6. Foster accountability	Encourage being responsible for behavior, most notably for within-treatment failures to remember or implement the lessons learned in prior sessions.
7. Maintain a focus on life outside of treatment	Stay informed about outside relationships and drinking behavior; emphasize the value of structured vocational activities.
8. Check in about the facts	Inquire about behaviors in a nonjudgmental way; address recovery setbacks directly, predictably, and systematically.

Note.   GPM-AUD = good psychiatric management of borderline personality disorder and alcohol use disorder.
Source.   Adapted from Gunderson and Links 2014.

Be Active, Not Reactive

Those with BPD who are interpersonally sensitive need to know you are committed. Remain active in your therapeutic interaction. Being quiet or passive or minimizing the patient's concerns can be seen as abandoning or hostile. Maintaining a nonjudgmental, highly respectful approach counteracts the shame and supports the patient's self-esteem, which is vital to them caring about what happens to themselves so that they can do the work of change.

Control struggles are common, so be prepared to sidestep them as a signal of splitting and prototypical dependence conflicts. Patients with

BPD often cope with intolerable and painful internal conflicts by externalizing them or shifting blame onto others. Keeping the conflict within the patient can help the patient exercise agency in making decisions independently. Ask questions that help the patient become more aware of these internal conflicts that they may be prone to externalizing into interpersonal conflict.

> *Patient*: It was horrible of me to drink so much at the holiday party. I guess they did say the limit was two drinks, and I had five. People don't understand how much I give to the company. I should be able to do what I want. Other people were drinking too, but my boss singled me out and told me to slow down.
>
> *Therapist*: I can tell this has been a painful experience for you. You wonder whether your boss was watching out for you, or whether it was your behavior and drinking that was the problem.

Patients with BPD express intense negative feelings that cause others to react in rescuing or rejecting ways, confirming the patient's negative or idealized expectations of others, which underlie maladaptive relational dynamics. Clinicians can recognize these enactments, which reinforce the patient's polarized view of themselves and others, and sidestep participating in them when possible. The more a clinician feels compelled to do something, the more they should think carefully about it first. Be receptive and invite patient disagreement. Express puzzlement to help foster reflection and remain active rather than reactive. Not overreacting allows you to become a model of thoughtful behavior and thinking before acting. This can be internalized and help the patient learn to communicate better with others. Overreacting with hospitalization or medication changes can be harmful. Slow patients down; pause them during narratives to allow them to clarify their feelings, desires, and sense of threat; and help them to find responses that others will better receive. You act as a container to "hold" patients and their projections of others.

Be Thoughtful

One of the goals (and mechanisms of change) in GPM is an increased ability for the patient to "think first." One of your main tasks as a treater is to facilitate thinking before acting, otherwise known as top-down regulation. You can model the value of being reflective, cautious, and curious by taking a *not knowing* stance (Bateman and Fonagy 2016). The attribution system in BPD is characterized by splitting (black or white;

all or nothing; good or bad). This is, in a way, reassuring, because it allows a sense of certainty, but such dichotomous views of oneself and others are rarely realistic or helpful. When clinicians display being comfortable with uncertainty and nuance, a role model of tolerance and interest in the unknown is helpful.

Thinking first involves helping the patient consider the pros and cons of their drinking and other behaviors. Be active while refraining from overly directive or insistent confrontations: "Is there more to this picture? Can you think of other reasons?" Invite reflection, thoughtfulness, and uncertainty rather than demanding it. Lessening extreme misattributions (e.g., that others have abandoned them or are acting maliciously) and learning to tolerate normal disappointment and hurt feelings in relationships will improve social functioning.

The Relationship Is Real as Well as Professional

Idealization of the clinician may be useful at the beginning of treatment, in that the patient is receptive to learning and recommendations. Over time, the relationship should become more real, allowing the patient to experience the value of a relationship that is "good enough" as opposed to perfect. Later, there may be grief once idealization diminishes and the clinician becomes a real person who has limitations, makes errors, or is simply not the hero or magic bullet patients with BPD hope for. Be ready to own your mistakes (e.g., "I must have misunderstood"). Acknowledging your mistakes sends the message that repair is possible in relationships. Making mistakes and repairing ruptures is a humanizing process, which provides a corrective experience for the patient, counteracts splitting, and enhances reality testing.

Selective self-disclosure can be used judiciously only if it benefits the patient, for example, "that would frustrate me too." Self-disclosure can help mitigate trust concerns, normalize feelings, make the relationship more authentic, and allow the patient to become more open in their discussions (Table 2–4). Also, careful self-disclosure can enlighten how the patient interaction pattern can impact others: "I want to help you, but it's hard for me to think when you scream at me."

Defining roles, boundaries, and expectations can help with the need for certainty, preserve the therapeutic relationship, and foster change. Discuss the importance of limits and how they can keep relationships healthy and sustainable over time. Addressing unrealistic expectations of yourself and others while conveying how this can be frustrating to the pa-

Table 2–4. Self-disclosure by clinicians in treating borderline personality disorder

Anonymity is a myth—what varies is the accuracy of a patient's perceptions; we affect this.

Ways that self-disclosure can help:

- To normalize feelings and beliefs that patients feel shamed by
- To encourage hope
- To establish authenticity
- To give permission to feel, say, act

Source.   Adapted from Gunderson and Links 2014.

tient can promote the understanding that the clinician is "not me." When this necessary disappointment happens in a soothing corrective relationship, the treater acts as a transitional object, and individualization can occur. Being warm and nonjudgmental, conveying acceptance when appropriate while promoting autonomous decision-making, and explaining your limitations and the impact the patient can have on you are all essential qualities to assist the patient in the therapeutic process.

Focus on Life Outside of Treatment

Interpersonal and situational triggers are the most significant predictors of self-destructive behavior (e.g., self-harm and binge drinking). Know what is happening in patients' primary relationships and work environment. Individuals with BPD and AUD have trouble making sense of emotion-laden experiences and interactions. The act of recognizing and labeling emotions aroused after a recent stressful interpersonal event can in itself lower their arousal and help them feel more connected to themselves (Lieberman et al. 2007). Enhancing realistic self-awareness allows patients to begin to make better sense of and reflect on experiences. In practical terms, the clinician can start this process by asking about what is happening in the patient's everyday life. Focusing on life outside treatment includes regularly checking in regarding their drinking behavior, as avoidance of this and similar topics is expected (see Chapter 3, "Integrating DDP and GPM").

The interpersonal hypersensitivity at the core of BPD can be buffered by having some sort of structured vocational activity, but full-time employment is often not a realistic goal in the short term for patients with BPD+AUD (Gregory 2022). Inform the patient about this and encourage them to take on responsibilities to gain mastery and a sense of valued contributions to their community. Encourage patients to take one step at a time: perhaps volunteer before paid work, part-time before full-time work, or an introductory academic class before a difficult one.

Change Is Expected

Inform patients that the course of BPD+AUD is one of gradual improvement, which depends on them. Educate them that you depend on them to take an active role in treatment. Patients should know that change is the goal and that you can assist them in achieving it, but the pathway to recovery can be arduous, and they must be comfortable with that decision. They need to proactively try the problem-solving strategies developed during sessions. Establish long-term goals to achieve recovery (e.g., acquire/maintain a full-time job and meaningful relationships, overcome alcohol-related problems), but stress that success is achieved by taking small steps at a time.

Ambivalence about change is to be expected. Patients with BPD+AUD remain ambivalent about independence and its necessary exposure to aloneness and increased responsibility. Relapses or self-harming behavior often return after a period of improvement. Balance giving validation that setbacks are common while holding patients accountable for self-defeating behaviors. Do not unrealistically insist on abstinence, because it can worsen coping, shame, and lying about relapses. It is important for patients to feel they can talk about any relapses into maladaptive behaviors. Self-discovery and learning about behavioral patterns take place as a process. Good treatment alliances can result in transforming chaotic expressions of ambivalence into tolerable and normal internal conflict.

Collaboratively evaluate whether signs of progress are being made in treatment (see "Assessing Progress" in Chapter 5). When treatment is not working, address everyone's contribution (yours and the patient's).

Foster Accountability

Foster a patient's sense of ownership of their problems and progress. Focus on what the patient can control and expect out of treatment. Responsibilities of the patient include staying in treatment, coming to appointments on time, actively participating in discussions, committing to recovery, taking medications, keeping themselves safe, and going to the emergency department when needed. Say that you depend on them to tell you what kind of help they need.

Having BPD results from an imbalance in stress in proportion to needed support, causing people with the disorder to experience developmental arrests in generating skills, building self-confidence, and understanding effective means of asking for help when they need it. When others (including the clinician) are idealized and perceived as all-powerful, patients feel helpless, expect the others to fix all problems, and become frustrated and resentful when those expectations are unmet. Clinicians can stay too long in an idealized position, by being too available and accommodating, in a way that reinforces the patient's stay in a passive role and covertly sustains a split that the patient is incapable and the clinician is all-capable. While validating difficulties, hold patients accountable for their actions. Expecting action and pushing for independence can convey confidence and respect to patients when communicated in a purposeful and genuine way. Such encouragements and expectations help set up patients to learn from their mistakes, build skills, and plan for better outcomes.

Check In About the Facts

Patients may be hesitant to disclose maladaptive behaviors such as substance use, self-harm, or excessive drinking out of shame, fear of judgment, and concerns about the potential consequences, such as hospitalization. The clinician must systematically inquire about these behaviors in a nonjudgmental manner and be attentive to any signs of clinical deterioration. Addressing problem behaviors directly, predictably, and systematically is the most effective way to accurately evaluate recovery progress and manage setbacks.

How Change Occurs

Patients with co-occurring BPD and AUD face overwhelming challenges from two sets of complex and disabling symptoms. The GPM clinician, informed by multiple perspectives (e.g., neurobiology, behavioral, psychodynamic) and a coherent model of BPD, can provide good-enough psychiatric management. By upholding the responsibilities of being a mental health professional trained to address both BPD and AUD, clinicians provide a credible and trustworthy foundation for a corrective therapeutic relationship on which more realistic appraisals of oneself and others and successful long-term stability can develop.

Corrective Experiences

People with BPD symptomatically have high expectations or idealization of others, which inevitably flips to frustration and devaluation. Listening,

Table 2–5. GPM's therapeutic processes

Process	Comment
Corrective experiences	Being listened to, cared for, and given realistic expectations are new experiences that improve trust, self-disclosure, capacity for closeness, and humility. Therapists who are trusting, reasonable, and reliable model qualities that can be internalized.
"Think first"	This process involves learning to think before acting, being aware of and able to label feelings, and thinking about one's experience and experiences within others (identifying feelings and motives)—called *mentalizing*.
Social and occupational rehabilitation	Encourage vocational stability as a means of regulating exposure to interpersonal intensity and instability.

Note.   GPM = good psychiatric management.
Source.   Adapted from Gunderson and Links 2014.

respecting the patient's point of view, being curious and authentic, acknowledging mistakes (i.e., real relationship), and collaboratively problem-solving provide a corrective framework that replaces unhealthy ways of relating (Table 2–5). The treater gradually transitions from an initial position of idealization and dependence toward being seen as a *not me* and a real individual. This therapeutic mode of relatedness for the patient is where differences of opinion can exist, people can disappoint each other, and relationships grow rather than end.

"Think First"

Impulsivity and emotion-processing deficits in BPD have neural substrates. The limbic system is hyperactivated and not counterbalanced by the prefrontal cortex. Brain regions associated with introspection, autobiographical memory, and recognizing and interpreting self and other mental states are altered in BPD (Gunderson et al. 2018; Ruocco and Carcone 2016), but these neural alterations can normalize with treatment (Iskric and Barkley-Levenson 2021).

GPM clinicians can use a variety of strategies to think before acting. Safety planning, "counting to 10," writing, talking, and planning ahead are examples of practical tools taught to patients so that they can delay acting on impulses. Both motivational interviewing and the consideration of pros and cons can structure comprehensive consideration of all sides of a situation before acting to diminish the instability that splitting causes in the behaviors of those with severe personality disorders. This also enhances what in dialectical behavioral therapy is called more dialectical thinking, rather than devolving to black-and-white tendencies. By serving as a good-enough model of judgment, the clinician encourages careful deliberation in a nonverbal and relational way.

Treaters can use autobiography and chain analyses to improve narrative coherence, establishing links between stressors, feelings, and maladaptive or self-destructive behaviors. Common to all effective therapies for BPD are efforts to help patients put into words their emotional experiences, make sense of them, and develop independence and authentic forms of relatedness, as well as tolerance and appreciation for multiple perspectives on the same experience both within oneself over time and between people in social interactions.

Social and Occupational Rehabilitation

Patients with BPD may initially use alcohol to cope with the emotional and relational turmoil typical of the disorder, but they end up on a self-perpetuating drinking loop, losing social connections and vocational functioning. Interpersonal hypersensitivity, driven by their insecurity over their capacity to manage on their own, influences those with BPD to become preoccupied with relationships over the more independent requirements of work or academic activities. The problem is that the overinvestment in relationships to which patients are inherently hypersensitive is destabilizing. As a comparison, patients with diabetes need to limit their intake of carbohydrates owing to their difficulty in metabolizing them. Similarly, those with BPD need to regulate their exposure to interpersonal intensity and uncertainty by forming a broader set of less intense and more structured relationships with roles and goals that are well defined. Vocational stability can foster a sense of agency, improve self-esteem, decrease shame, and buffer insecurities arising from relationship setbacks. Clinicians need to emphasize the choice to "get a life"; otherwise, treatment with dependent patients can easily become regressive (i.e., increasing dependence). The goal is for the treatment to become obsolete as the patient improves and develops better ways to use their time.

Conclusion

BPD and AUD patients have a difficult time processing social information and recognizing their emotions, which leads to, at first, seemingly unpredictable clinical decompensation. The IHS model explains this phenomenon and is useful in providing psychoeducation to patients and families and anchoring clinical interventions. In addition, having in mind the basic principles of good psychiatric care helps ground clinicians during turbulent times so that they do not lose sight of the basic treatment goals and can organize interventions effectively around a shared framework. A coherent formulation of symptoms and a manualized approach are common features of empirically validated treatments for BPD. Additionally, GPM uses the medical model, which can reduce stigma and aid in navigating the complex scenario of challenging comorbidities and establishing priorities. With this set of tools, the clinician, who provides a professional but also real relationship, lays the foundation for a corrective experience, in which the patient learns how to take the steps toward recovery in a trusting and collaborative environment.

3

Integrating Dynamic Deconstructive Psychotherapy Into Good Psychiatric Management

Robert J. Gregory, M.D.
Lois W. Choi-Kain, M.D., M.Ed.

Dynamic deconstructive psychotherapy (DDP) was originally developed for more challenging cases of borderline personality disorder (BPD), especially those accompanied by co-occurring substance use disorders (Gregory and Remen 2008). The first randomized controlled trial of DDP was for individuals with co-occurring BPD and alcohol use disorder (AUD). Compared with optimized community care, DDP demonstrated superior outcomes across a wide range of outcomes, with sustained effects noted for alcohol and drug use 18 months after treatment ended (Gregory et al. 2008; 2010).

According to DDP theory, drinking can serve multiple functions for an individual with BPD. It can reduce social inhibitions, dampen anxiety through direct and indirect effects on the central nervous system, help block out awareness of painful emotions, and provide euphoria and self-soothing through activation of the attachment system (Gregory 2019; Gregory and Remen 2008). The use of alcohol (and many other drugs) provides an effective short-term solution for many of the challenges faced by those with BPD, and it is no wonder that two-thirds have co-occurring substance use disorders (Zanarini et al. 2004).

Of course, the short-term benefits of drinking come at a terrible price. Frequent intoxication leads to impaired relationships, occupational dysfunction, legal difficulties, and low self-esteem. Prolonged withdrawal from alcohol exacerbates underlying anxiety, dysphoria, and mood reactivity. Perhaps most importantly, drinking perpetuates a person's lifelong coping pattern of disconnection from their self and their experiences, as well as disconnection from others, and blocks the opportunity to form authentic relationships. Disconnection leads to a sense of emptiness and being stuck alone with overwhelming pain, thereby contributing to suicide risk.

Treatment with DDP aims to help an individual lead a connected life. It involves weekly psychotherapy over 12 months through distinct treatment stages, beginning with establishing a clear framework and judgment-free space for sharing and reflection; fostering the patient's autonomous decision-making and working through ambivalence; facilitating the patient's ability to put day-to-day emotionally laden experiences into words and label their emotions, and opening up new perspectives on those experiences; developing a capacity for authentic relatedness by providing novel experiences in here-and-now patient-therapist interactions that open up new possibilities for relatedness; and finally, mourning painful realities, working toward self-acceptance, and making peace with themselves.

Principles of Dynamic Deconstructive Psychotherapy

To achieve advanced competency in DDP, a trainee must bring at least two patients through all the treatment stages while receiving weekly case consultation from an advanced competency therapist. This is a substantial investment in training for clinicians, and it is not always feasible to provide weekly psychotherapy in medical and psychiatric settings. Even without implementation of weekly DDP, however, many of its principles can be usefully applied in the good psychiatric management of patients with BPD+AUD (GPM-AUD). These seven principles are summarized in the remainder of the chapter (Table 3–1). These distilled core principles overlap with elements of GPM-AUD as a basis of integration between the two approaches.

Table 3-1.   Seven principles of DDP

Principle	Summary
Judgment-free zone	Counteract the negative cycle of criticism and defensiveness in individuals with AUD by providing a nonjudgmental environment, promoting patient autonomy, and fostering reflective thinking for personal growth and understanding.
Build narratives	Facilitate emotion labeling and autobiographical memory in individuals with BPD + AUD to enhance higher-level emotion processing, relieve heightened arousal and cravings, promote reflection, and expedite recovery, while fostering self-development.
Support self-esteem	Promote self-esteem and confront denial in individuals with AUD by medicalizing their drinking, reframing relapse as a chronic medical condition. This alleviates guilt and motivates ongoing engagement in treatment and recovery.
Check in regularly	Proactively address avoidance and misattribution in individuals with AUD by regularly assessing their drinking behavior, even in the face of difficulty and shame, to ensure accurate evaluation and provide balanced education on the impact of alcohol on mental health.
Inform, not advise	Limit advice-giving to avoid negative outcomes and instead offer psychoeducation as consultants, respecting patient autonomy in decision-making.
Integrate splitting	Explore both positive and negative aspects of drinking while addressing polarized perspectives, anger, and shame to treat dissociative splitting that people with BPD + AUD rely on as a coping mechanism. Splitting undermines the capacity for balanced decisions about drinking.
Build authentic relatedness	Address competing dependency needs and fears within patients by working in a professional and therefore predictable but genuine fashion in setting boundaries, fostering collaboration, promoting authentic disagreement, supporting autonomy, and checking for ambivalence to enhance the therapeutic alliance.

Note.   AUD = alcohol use disorder; BPD = borderline personality disorder; DDP = dynamic deconstructive psychotherapy.

Judgment-Free Zone

Although it's not always obvious to either the clinician or the patient, individuals with AUD universally struggle with low self-esteem and interpersonal sensitivity. Underlying shame is defended against through grandiosity, leading clinicians to communicate—directly or indirectly—to patients with AUD to "get out of my emergency room!" Meanwhile, patients use denial and blame of others for their difficulties. Their assumption of the victim role and their refusal to take any responsibility for their difficulties push our clinician buttons very strongly, making us want to forcibly break through the denial. It is tempting for us to say things like: "Don't you think that showing up drunk for work played a large role in your getting fired?" "It is likely that your being drunk and irritable was the cause of your boyfriend leaving you." "You have no one to blame but yourself for drinking and driving!"

Such forceful assertions can help a clinician to feel more empowered in the absence of control over the situation but are likely to generate one of two reactions from the patient: either defensiveness or hopelessness.

To sidestep this pattern, even when a clinician is feeling frustrated, they can refrain from criticism or judgments and instead support patient autonomy. At the beginning of treatment, a clinician can tell the patient:

> I want this to be a judgment-free zone. You are free to share or bring up anything you like with me, and you will not be judged for it.

Then the clinician needs to follow through when tested. Open the door to the denial system, instead of pushing the patient through it, by asking questions with curiosity, like: "Can you think of any other reasons that you might have been fired?" "Does part of you blame yourself for your boyfriend leaving you?" "What is it like to wake up and not remember what happened when you drove home the night before?" These caring, curious, and nonjudgmental inquiries seem easy in theory but can be incredibly difficult when you are in the room with a patient and are overcome with negative emotions and urges to take control of the situation. Clinicians need to be in a cognitively and emotionally steady place to do this hard work. A nonjudgmental approach facilitates more flexible, nuanced, and reflective thinking to move patients forward in their ability to understand themselves more clearly. The judgment-free zone of DDP enables optimal consideration of oneself in interaction with the world—that is, one's efforts to cope and foster relationships with others.

Build Narratives

Help the patient begin to connect with their emotions and experiences by having them talk about their recent emotionally laden interpersonal experiences or relapses, create a specific sequence of interactions or events, and label their emotions. Individuals with BPD+AUD have an impaired emotion-processing system characterized by atrophy or dysfunction of many of the higher-level brain regions responsible for remembering emotion-laden interactions and putting them into words as a coherent narrative (Schulze et al. 2016). This difficulty with higher-level emotion processing contributes to identity disturbance, dissociation, and inability to gain perspective and self-soothe. In contrast, the subcortical regions, especially the amygdala and ventral striatum, become hyperactivated in response to emotional stimuli, leading to anxiety, hyperarousal, and impulsive pleasure-seeking or dependent attachment-seeking for self-soothing.

One of the goals of treatment is therefore to remediate the higher-level emotion-processing pathways through repeated practice, much like physical and occupational therapies remediate impaired motor neuron pathways. Neuroscience research suggests that the simple act of labeling an emotion, such as anger or shame, can decrease amygdala activation and physiological arousal (Lieberman et al. 2007).

In practical terms, when a patient comes to our office stating that they have been more depressed and anxious, we can ask them questions, such as: "When did it start?" "Had you been drinking that day or the day before?" "What else had been going on that day?" "So, your boyfriend told you that? Tell me what happened in the conversation." "What emotions did you experience when he said that?" Typically, patients will respond to that last question by saying "anxious," "confused," or "upset," which just indicates that the patient was in a state of arousal but does not inform us of the underlying emotion that caused the arousal. Alternatively, they will respond with an attribution, instead of an emotion, such as, "She just wanted to hurt me." Most typically, the underlying emotions that are driving the arousal and subsequent craving for alcohol are a combination of anger and shame. If the clinician is able to help the patient to acknowledge and label those emotions, the patient often can find a sense of relief from lowered arousal and will be less likely to go into hyperdrive the next time a similar event happens; rather, they will start to build some reflective space. To accelerate their recovery, a diary card or journaling can be used between sessions to practice connecting with their emotions and experiences. This process of building narratives converges with GPM-AUD's emphasis on building autobiography as a bridge to a more solidified sense of self. Most clinicians already foster such discussions to understand their patients better; ultimately, it kindles a greater self-understanding on the part of the patient, as well.

Support Self-Esteem

How do we support self-esteem while challenging the denial system? How do we inject hope when we ourselves are feeling helpless and hopeless? The denial system maintains self-esteem by minimizing the severity of the drinking, shifting responsibility onto others, and creating a fantasy of control over drinking. As comedian W.C. Fields quipped, "Don't say you can't swear off drinking; it's easy. I've done it a thousand times!" Those with AUD are likely to say something very similar about their drinking, but not get the humor of their statements. The CAGE screener (cut down, annoyed, guilty, eye-opener; see Appendix E) assesses the denial system with the following prompt: "Have you ever tried to cut down on your drinking?"

Step 1 of the Alcoholics Anonymous (AA) Twelve Steps involves admitting powerlessness over drinking behavior. On the surface, this seems like the worst possible intervention to make for someone who is already blaming others for all their problems; it gets them off the hook! Paradoxically, Step 1 is the most difficult step for someone with AUD to buy into, because it cuts through their denial system. It is also the single most important step in recovery, since it provides an alternative to denial as a means of supporting self-esteem and relieving the enormous burden of guilt and shame. If one has an illness that involves uncontrolled drinking, then there is no need to feel ashamed over drinking behavior; treatment becomes the focus.

In practical terms, when a patient shamefacedly admits to us that they messed up and got drunk last night, we can undercut their denial, inject hope, and support their self-esteem by medicalizing and normalizing their drinking, linking it to Step 1. Here is an example of a useful intervention in that circumstance:

> Relapse is nothing to be ashamed of or embarrassed by. Alcoholism is a chronic relapsing medical condition over which you have limited control. That's what Step 1 of AA tells us, that we don't have control over our drinking; and if we don't have control over it, then there is no more shame in relapse than there is in having a heart attack or stroke. Many people forget that fact and beat themselves up every time they relapse and give up on themselves and recovery. But the important thing is to get right back in the saddle after relapse. Even though you have limited control over your drinking, what you do have complete control over is deciding to get in treatment and stay in treatment. And if you do that, the relapses will become less frequent and severe over time.

Other ways to support self-esteem are to highlight positive attributes and be careful to phrase drinking problems as a medical issue, rather than a moral issue. For instance, the clinician can state (if true): "You are clearly an intelligent and insightful person and have the potential for great success in life once your illness is brought under better control."

Also, clinicians need to be on guard for moralistic verbiage that tends to slip into the lexicon of addiction with terms such as "clean" instead of "abstinent," or "alcohol abuse" instead of "alcohol use disorder." Often patients with AUD will accuse their clinicians of not trusting them to stay abstinent. The clinician can move the illness from the moral to the medical realm by responding:

> You have a chronic relapsing illness that is outside your control. It's like someone on the beach saying, "Trust me, I can swim," when there is a tsunami behind them. Relapse is not a matter of trust!

Check In Regularly

One aspect of the denial system is avoidance and misattribution. It is very common for an AUD patient to avoid telling their clinician about their increased drinking behavior and to attribute worsening psychiatric symptoms or functioning to something other than drinking. Patients may be quite definite about the cause of their worsening symptoms, and that it has nothing to do with their drinking. They may state that they are drinking more because of their worsened stress and mental state, not the other way around. Likewise, when they start to feel better, they are likely to attribute the improvement to a change in medication or decreased stressors, rather than a reduction in drinking.

It is important for clinicians to regularly check in with their patients regarding their drinking behavior. Clinicians do not necessarily have to ask about drinking every week, but it is important to do so regularly, especially when there is evidence of clinical worsening. This can be done in a matter-of-fact manner—for instance: "Have you been drinking more lately?"

Checking in may be harder than it sounds. As clinicians, we empathically sense that this is a difficult and shame-ridden topic for the patient; often we mutually avoid talking about it. Clinicians need to be aware of their own hesitancy and ask the difficult screening question.

Alternatively, clinicians can check in regarding worsening drinking behavior by administering brief self-rated screening questions on a monthly or quarterly basis. The screening does not have to be extensive, because the drinking problem has already been established. Follow-up screening can be as simple as a single question adapted from the Addiction Severity Index, such as, "In the past month, how many days have you had at least four or five drinks containing alcohol (wine, beer, or liquor)?" (McLellan et al. 1992). (The index states four drinks for women and five for men.) A more formal tool is the three-item AUDIT-C (Alcohol Use Disorders Identification Test-Concise), which uses multiple choice questions to quantify the frequency and quantity of drinking behavior and has shown good sensitivity and specificity for detecting problem drinking (Bush et al. 1998). See Appendix E for a list of screening instruments.

If patients attribute their increased drinking behavior to increased stress, clinicians need to provide education in a matter-of-fact and balanced manner about how drinking may indeed be a stress reliever while it is in their system, but that it actually can worsen their anxiety and depression for up to 2–3 days after the alcohol leaves their system (see example in the next section for phrasing).

Inform, Not Advise

Although giving advice or direction is a common GPM intervention, it should be used sparingly with patients having BPD+AUD. For many such patients, greater directiveness can lead to worse outcomes (Karno and Longabaugh, 2005). They often react to advice by disowning personal responsibility for their recovery through either regressive compliance or getting into a control struggle. If we find ourselves in a control struggle with a patient, the session is heading in the wrong direction and is unlikely to be helpful.

Individuals with BPD+AUD have a strong desire for autonomy and control and resent being told what to do. Also, if they draw us into a control struggle, they avoid facing the painful reality of their drinking behavior. In other words, they create external conflicts as a way to avoid internal conflicts. They may say, "I'm fine with my drinking; you're the one who has a problem with it, not me!" Paradoxically, the outward rebellion suggests a desire for independence, but on the backdrop of reckless behavior, it invites overinvolvement and restores dependence on others or the system. The patient then enters a vicious cycle that undermines self-reliance and autonomy.

Complicating this situation is that patients with AUD are able to push clinician buttons in many ways. We may become so concerned about our patients' dangerous and erratic behaviors, feeling helpless and frustrated, that we get drawn into a more directive stance and make invalidating comments or questions. The rule of thumb is to keep the conflict within the patient!

Does that mean that we should walk on tiptoe when it comes to the harmful effects of drinking? Not at all! It is the clinician's duty to provide psychoeducation regarding the effects of drinking on health and functioning and to render an opinion regarding the effects that heavy alcohol consumption may have. Psychoeducation is inherent in both DDP and GPM-AUD. But it is more effective to do so in the role of a consultant, helping patients to weigh the pros and cons, and respecting that only the patient can decide what is best.

It is problematic to state:

> Drinking is causing your anxiety and depression, and you simply need to quit.

It is better to psychoeducate:

> Even though drinking can be helpful for anxiety for the brief time it's in our bodies, it gets metabolized out of our bodies very quickly, and withdrawal can last for days. Even moderate amounts of drinking can affect how anxious, reactive, and depressed we are for the next 2 to 3 days.

or advise:

> I believe that your drinking is significantly contributing to your anxiety and depression. I understand that the brief benefits from drinking may still be worth it for you, but it's my job to let you know about the potential downsides as well, so that you can weigh the risks and benefits and decide what is best for you.

Both DDP and GPM-AUD promote realistic or frank conversation that is easily grasped but may provoke strong emotions for those who are interpersonally and emotionally hypersensitive. Combining frank, objective, clinical perspectives with sparing advice promotes the type of agency required for durable change in both alcohol use and personality functioning. GPM-AUD advocates for a professional but real relationship in which symptoms are discussed in a medically objective, realistic way.

Integrate Splitting

Along with drinking, individuals with BPD+AUD disconnect from their experiences with dissociative splitting. Splitting involves polarized and poorly integrated emotions, motivations, and beliefs about oneself and others. Splitting, when combined with interpersonal sensitivity, accounts for the rapid mood shifts and mood reactivity that characterize BPD. Patients can appear depressed and needy in the emergency department and then angry and defiant when they are admitted to a psychiatric unit. These sudden shifts from one setting to another, or from one interaction to another, can lead to polarized "split" attitudes in the clinical staff caring for them, and may create an impression in some of the staff members that the patients are just being manipulative.

Splitting also reinforces the denial system and makes it particularly difficult for individuals with BPD+AUD to make balanced decisions regarding their drinking behavior, which likely contributes to their relatively poor prognosis (Zanarini et al. 2004). They are likely to describe drinking as all-good or all-bad, with very little integration of those two perspectives. For example, they might state: "Drinking is the only thing that helps me be myself; it helps me to unwind and be more relaxed in social situations." Alternatively, they might state: "Drinking is a nasty habit and doesn't do anything good for me." To help patients make an informed choice over their drinking, it is necessary for clinicians to help their patients explore both sides of the split in an even-handed manner: what they like about drinking, as well as what they don't like or are concerned about. As mentioned earlier in "Inform, Not Advise," clinicians can provide psychoeducation about harmful effects or render clinical opinions about possible harms, but this must be done in a way that does not engender a control struggle.

Splitting is not restricted to drinking behavior. It may also lead to polarized and poorly integrated perspectives of the self and others as being all-good or all-bad. Patients may have a polarized and poorly integrated sense of personal responsibility, feeling totally responsible for every bad thing that ever happened to them, alternating with feeling a total lack of ownership or personal responsibility. An excessive sense of personal responsibility is accompanied by shame, depression, or suicidality; a lack of personal responsibility is accompanied by anger, entitlement, and suspiciousness. Anger and shame are therefore the two critical emotions that underlie much of the anxiety, maladaptive behaviors, and chaotic relationships of patients with BPD+AUD and are the key emotions to help patients verbalize and acknowledge when building narratives. As a general rule, the more strongly a patient expresses a certain emotion or belief, the more likely it is that the opposite emotion or belief is also present but is being split off and not acknowledged. The clinician therefore tries to help bring these split-off attributes into consciousness.

For example, if the patient says how angry they are that their spouse unjustly criticizes them, the clinician might respond:

> Even though you know it's not true, I wonder if part of you feels that you deserve the criticism?

If the patient responds affirmatively, the clinician can ask:

> What is the emotion that goes along with the thought that you deserve the criticism?

In DDP theory, splitting is seen more broadly as polarized and conflicting attributions within the self. These attributions include *value (idealization vs. devaluation)*, *agency (victim vs. perpetrator)*, and *motivation (autonomy vs. dependence)* (Table 3–2) Alcohol use provides a stabilizing solution to the chaos and anxiety caused by these conflicting and poorly integrated attributions and reduces the potential vulnerability and risk

Table 3–2. Polarized and conflicting attributions within the self

Attribute	Polarities
Value	Idealization vs. devaluation
Agency	Victim vs. perpetrator
Motivation	Autonomy vs. dependence

for rejection in relationships. Drinking becomes the idealized object that can never disappoint (value). Others are blamed for any negative consequences of the drinking behavior, so there is no further internal conflict regarding agency, either. Drinking solves the conflicting motivations as well, by providing a sense of closeness and comfort and also a sense of empowerment and control. In Winnicott's terms, drinking becomes a transitional object providing a substitute for mother's caring, while also providing a sense of autonomy through the fantasy of control. Drinking therefore is very difficult to give up, especially for those with interpersonal instability and intolerance of being alone.

Splitting is the essential destabilizing force behind GPM-AUD's interpersonal hypersensitivity model (see Figure 2–1). In GPM, the traditional components of splitting emphasize phases of idealization followed by devaluation, as a tendency associated with need-fear attachment dynamics, which destabilizes relationships due to the poorly integrated attributions that come from unprocessed emotional and interpersonal experiences. GPM takes a descriptive approach to splitting to provide an organizing framework for understanding the interpersonal instabilities as arising from the patient's internal insecurity, and their reaction to that insecurity, which causes them to first idealize others and then feel easily threatened by their unavailability. When people with BPD depend heavily on others to meet their needs in an ideal way, realistic problems inevitably threaten their unrealistic expectations. In the face of these inevitable interpersonal disappointments, they lash out in anger that their all-good relationship is crumbling. This sort of aggression drives others to angrily reject the person with BPD or withdraw out of fear, confusion, and helplessness. Alcohol use can temporarily provide a resolution of this prototypic need-fear dilemma by enhancing a false sense of self-sufficiency while also dampening painful emotions in a way that diminishes the need for support.

Combining these two angles on the splitting problem in BPD enables clinicians and patients to share a framework to understand how splitting destabilizes relationships, manifests symptoms of BPD, and generates the urge to drink. Both models encourage processing and making sense of how symptomatic episodes arise. BPD symptoms and alcohol use influence the patient's unstable sense of self and relationships; the two frameworks help reduce black-and-white thinking or polarized attributions, emotional reactivity, and destructive behavior aimed inward or outward.

Build Authentic Relatedness

A more insidious form of splitting gets played out in the relationship between patients with BPD+AUD and their care providers. One form of splitting is in regard to motivation. Patients with BPD+AUD often have strong dependency needs, but they also have fears of vulnerability in close relationships and the need to remain autonomous and in control.

These conflicting and poorly integrated interpersonal motivations create a push-pull quality to relationships with care providers that gets played out through drinking behaviors. Drinking can create a euphoric sense of closeness and belonging through activation of the μ opioid receptors in the ventral striatum, which is part of the reward and attachment systems in the brain (Moles et al. 2004). Drinking may therefore meet attachment needs and sometimes serve as a substitute for close relationships. For individuals with BPD who have strong dependency needs in combination with fears of vulnerability in close relationships, drinking offers the perfect solution. It provides the sense of closeness without the vulnerability. Through the use of the denial system, alcohol provides a relationship over which they have a fantasy of control (see earlier section, "Support Self-Esteem").

The way this dynamic can play out in the clinician-patient relationship is for patients to desire closeness, advice, and direction from the clinician, but then react with increased drinking behavior when these desires are met because of their wish for autonomy and their fear of vulnerability. Increased drinking behavior during treatment therefore can be a marker for increased ambivalence regarding the treatment and the clinician-patient relationship. The challenge for clinicians is to meet some of the patient's attachment needs for caring and concern, but also to limit the patient's sense of vulnerability and to support autonomous decision-making. In this way, the patient can learn to tolerate the closeness of the clinician-patient relationship without resorting to drinking

Table 3–3. Strategies to balance attachment needs and autonomy

Strategy	Steps
Clear boundaries, roles, and expectations	Specify these early in treatment and seek agreement from the patient. The clearer the limits of the clinician-patient relationship, the less the patient will need to test those limits. Three key expectations to have of the patient are as follows: 1) work toward health and recovery; 2) actively participate in treatment; and 3) do not engage in hostility toward the clinician.
Agreed-on goals and tasks	To strengthen the alliance, develop goals and tasks in collaboration with the patient to support self-agency and autonomous motivation.
A "target" on the therapist	Paint a target on yourself to encourage disagreement. This tells the patient that they are free to be authentic in their relationship with you (within the limits that you set at the beginning). When there is no disagreement, there is no authenticity.
Support for autonomous decision-making	Support the patient's autonomous decision-making regarding values and life choices, including decisions regarding their drinking behavior. This may be very difficult when you disagree with their choices.
Frequently discuss and normalize ambivalence toward the treatment and clinician	Ambivalence toward treatment and recovery is normal. The more a patient is able to verbalize their ambivalence, the less likely they will act it out through no-shows or increased drinking.

and may develop a capacity for authentic relatedness. Some specific strategies are outlined in Table 3–3.

Conclusion

Individuals with BPD+AUD are stuck in a lifelong coping pattern of disconnection from themselves and other people through the use of drinking, denial, and dissociative splitting. DDP aims to reverse this pattern of disconnection by helping patients to build narratives of emotion-laden experiences, reduce denial and dissociative splitting, and develop authentic relatedness in the clinician-patient relationship. A key to success is clinician self-awareness and the ability to contain any buttons that the patient may push, to stay within a therapeutic frame. Ideally, the main focus of treatment is helping the patient to connect to their experiences through exploration of recent emotion-laden interactions, rather than focusing exclusively on reducing drinking behavior. But drinking behavior should not be ignored and should be asked about regularly and explored in the context of emotions and interpersonal relationships. Drinking is viewed as part of the patient's former coping strategy of disconnection, and increased drinking is therefore a marker of ambivalence toward the treatment and the treatment relationship. A "side effect" of creating a connected life is less desire to drink.

These central facets of DDP—the only approach found to be effective expressly for BPD co-occurring with AUD—can be adapted to a generalist psychiatric management of patients with BPD+AUD. The facets outlined in this chapter tailor GPM-AUD's practical basic approach to addressing alcohol use problems. By incorporating these elements of DDP, an effective treatment for BPD+AUD, those practicing GPM-AUD can tailor their approach to proactively treat alcohol use and enhance opportunities for corrective experiences that might repair the shame and mistrust that reinforce the two disorders.

4

Making the Diagnosis

Rocco Iannucci, M.D.
Grace Murray, B.A.
Stephen Conway, M.D.

Comprehensive assessment remains the foundation of all treatment. A shared understanding between patient and therapist of therapeutic problems and agreed-on goals will foster collaborative clinical work and a productive relationship. Clinicians may experience anxiety about making or sharing a diagnosis of borderline personality disorder (BPD) or alcohol use disorder (AUD) for fear that it will be poorly received by the patient, or that it may be experienced as stigmatizing. Yet evidence consistently demonstrates that this process—naming the diagnosis—is itself therapeutic. Clear communication of an accurate diagnosis provides education and hope, sets the stage for treatment engagement, clarifies goals, and informs the selection of treatment options. A collaborative assessment process between patient and clinician, incorporating strategies to assess readiness and enhance patient motivation, promotes patient engagement and agency in choosing among treatment options. Treatment engagement requires joint effort by both the patient and the clinician to identify symptoms, establish diagnoses, and provide relevant normative feedback and psychoeducation about treatment options.

Why Make the Diagnoses?

Diagnostic labels are limited in how well they describe a given person's struggles and strengths, but they can be useful in guiding treatment decisions. Formal psychiatric diagnoses are an important component of a biopsychosocial formulation. In addition, most clinical trials of medication and psychotherapeutic treatments rely on established diagnoses based on DSM-5-TR (American Psychiatric Association 2022) and ICD-11 (World Health Organization 2022) to select subjects. Hence, evidence-based treatment must be grounded in a comprehensive assessment that includes formal diagnosis.

Awareness that a patient has BPD can also help a clinician to respond appropriately to common interpersonal dynamics that arise in treatment. Without knowledge of the diagnosis, a clinician may respond with surprise or countertherapeutic interventions, such as punitive or avoidant behavior. Given the interpersonal hypersensitivity that is often at the core of BPD symptoms, combined with the role of shame as both a consequence and risk factor for substance use, it is especially important to foster an open, nonjudgmental dynamic between the patient and the treater (Luoma et al. 2019). Frank diagnostic disclosure and psychoeducation can medicalize the symptoms, separate diagnosis from identity, and break the cycle of stigma and shame (Aviram et al. 2006). Some research shows that active and agential communication with psychiatrists is associated with lower levels of self-stigma and shame and higher levels of self-responsibility in consumers of mental health treatment (Hamann et al. 2017).

Diagnostic disclosure in the good psychiatric management (GPM) model aims to support the patient's agency by involving them collaboratively in the diagnosis and conveying realistic optimism regarding the expected course and available treatments for the diagnosis. The patient can gain a valuable perspective on their own behavior with an understanding of the syndrome criteria, severity, community epidemiology, and their individual patterns of expressing diagnostic components. In the GPM approach, naming and explicit discussion of interpersonal hypersensitivity not only helps a patient make sense of their past experiences, but it also facilitates helpful, clinical discussion of such challenges when they arise in treatment (Gunderson and Links 2014). Likewise, evidence-based treatment of AUD considers development of the disorder (genetic loading in the family, alcohol exposure in the family and community, stress and other mental health factors increasing vulnerability to problem drinking) and examination of the progression of AUD's severity (quantity/frequency over time, loss of control, health consequences) in discussing safety, treatment needs, and what interventions are most likely to be effective for drinking reduction goals. Because many presenting with at-risk alcohol use or AUD will be interested in reduced alcohol consumption rather than abstinence, personalizing goals and outlining a structured, evidence-based plan to achieve those goals will be most effective (Hasin et al. 2017).

Diagnostic Criteria for AUD and BPD

Symptoms of AUD can be categorized into four domains: physiological dependence (ethanol tolerance and alcohol withdrawal syndrome during abstinence), cravings and mental preoccupation with drinking, continued use despite negative consequences, and problems controlling use (drinking greater quantities or more frequently than intended, failed attempts to cut back) (Box 4–1 and Table 4–1). There is no hierarchy of symptoms, with all criteria being applied equally. Those experiencing two or more DSM-5-TR symptom criteria within a 12-month period are diagnosed with AUD. Based on total number of symptom criteria, the severity of AUD is determined to be mild, moderate, or severe (American Psychiatric Association 2022) (Figure 4–1).

Box 4-1. Alcohol Use Disorder

A. A problematic pattern of alcohol use leading to clinically significant impairment or distress, as manifested by at least two of the following, occurring within a 12-month period:

1. Alcohol is often taken in larger amounts or over a longer period than was intended.
2. There is a persistent desire or unsuccessful efforts to cut down or control alcohol use.
3. A great deal of time is spent in activities necessary to obtain alcohol, use alcohol, or recover from its effects.
4. Craving, or a strong desire or urge to use alcohol.
5. Recurrent alcohol use resulting in a failure to fulfill major role obligations at work, school, or home.
6. Continued alcohol use despite having persistent or recurrent social or interpersonal problems caused or exacerbated by the effects of alcohol.

7. Important social, occupational, or recreational activities are given up or reduced because of alcohol use.

8. Recurrent alcohol use in situations in which it is physically hazardous.

9. Alcohol use is continued despite knowledge of having a persistent or recurrent physical or psychological problem that is likely to have been caused or exacerbated by alcohol.

10. Tolerance, as defined by either of the following:

    a. A need for markedly increased amounts of alcohol to achieve intoxication or desired effect.

    b. A markedly diminished effect with continued use of the same amount of alcohol.

11. Withdrawal, as manifested by either of the following:

    a. The characteristic withdrawal syndrome for alcohol (refer to Criteria A and B of the criteria set for alcohol withdrawal).

    b. Alcohol (or a closely related substance, such as a benzodiazepine) is taken to relieve or avoid withdrawal symptoms.

Source.   Reprinted from American Psychiatric Association: *Diagnostic and Statistical Manual of Mental Disorders*, 5th Edition, Text Revision. Washington, DC, American Psychiatric Association, 2022. Copyright © 2022 American Psychiatric Association. Used with permission.

BPD is a disorder of dysregulation across four domains: cognition, affect, behavior, and interpersonal relationships. Specific symptoms include dissociation and stress-related psychosis (cognitive); angry outbursts and moodiness (affective); self-injurious behavior and impulsive behavior, including reckless driving or spending (behavioral); and stormy relationships and engaging in efforts to avoid abandonment (interpersonal). As in AUD, all symptoms are weighted equally when assessing BPD, with five or more symptoms sufficient to make the diagnosis (Box 4–2) (American Psychiatric Association 2022).

Table 4–1. Criteria for alcohol use disorder (see Box 4–1)

Diagnostic criteria	Examples
Physiological dependence • Greater amounts of alcohol are required to achieve the desired effect • Typical symptoms of alcohol withdrawal occur during abstinent periods, and alcohol may be used to relieve them	• Switching from beer to a similar volume of higher-proof liquor because the previous intake "doesn't do anything anymore" • Experiencing medical symptoms such as anxiety, sweating, hypertension, tremulousness, seizure, or hallucination after abrupt cessation of alcohol use (severe alcohol withdrawal is a potentially life-threatening condition)
Preoccupation • Cravings or urges are experienced when not drinking • A substantial amount of time is spent getting, using, or recovering from the effects of alcohol	• Having cravings or urges to drink between drinking episodes • Spending substantial time planning how, when, and where to consume alcohol
Continued alcohol use despite negative consequences • Leads to role impairment at work, school, or home • Leads to reduction or loss of important activities • Continues despite adverse consequences • Continues despite adverse social or interpersonal consequences • Alcohol is repeatedly used in situations where it is dangerous	• Continuing to drink heavily despite being aware that alcohol use is causing absenteeism at work or marital strife • Intoxication while pregnant, while solely responsible for a dependent, or while driving
Loss of control over use • Alcohol is used in greater quantities or duration than intended • Inability to stop or reduce alcohol use	• Planning a "quick drink" but remaining at a bar until closing • Repeatedly resolving to cut down or stop alcohol use, while being unable to achieve or sustain this goal

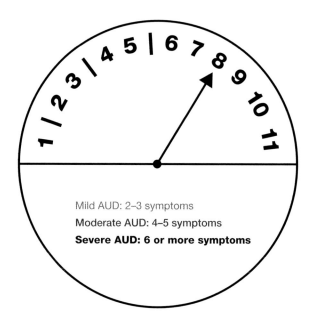

Figure 4–1.   Severity of AUD symptoms.

Note.   AUD = alcohol use disorder.

Box 4-2.   Borderline Personality Disorder

A pervasive pattern of instability of interpersonal relationships, self-image, and affects, and marked impulsivity, beginning by early adulthood and present in a variety of contexts, as indicated by five (or more) of the following:

1. Frantic efforts to avoid real or imagined abandonment. (**Note:** Do not include suicidal or self-mutilating behavior covered in Criterion 5.)
2. A pattern of unstable and intense interpersonal relationships characterized by alternating between extremes of idealization and devaluation.
3. Identity disturbance: markedly and persistently unstable self-image or sense of self.
4. Impulsivity in at least two areas that are potentially self-damaging (e.g., spending, sex, substance abuse, reckless driving, binge eating). (**Note:** Do not include suicidal or self-mutilating behavior covered in Criterion 5.)
5. Recurrent suicidal behavior, gestures, or threats, or self-mutilating behavior.

6. Affective instability due to a marked reactivity of mood (e.g., intense episodic dysphoria, irritability, or anxiety usually lasting a few hours and only rarely more than a few days).
7. Chronic feelings of emptiness.
8. Inappropriate, intense anger or difficulty controlling anger (e.g., frequent displays of temper, constant anger, recurrent physical fights).
9. Transient, stress-related paranoid ideation or severe dissociative symptoms.

Source. Reprinted from American Psychiatric Association: *Diagnostic and Statistical Manual of Mental Disorders*, 5th Edition, Text Revision. Washington, DC, American Psychiatric Association, 2022. Copyright © 2022 American Psychiatric Association. Used with permission.

GPM conceptualizes BPD as primarily a disorder of interpersonal hypersensitivity. Individuals with BPD may cycle through connected, threatened, alone, and despairing states (see Figures 2–1 and 2–2), and specific symptoms become salient in each state. For example, when an individual with BPD feels *connected* in their interpersonal relationships, they may be idealizing but hypersensitive to rejection. If they become *threatened* in their interpersonal relationships, they may be more likely to experience dissociation and paranoia related to their relationships. See Chapter 10 for more information on how an individual may transition between these states and the relevant symptomatology. See later section "Common Problems" for a discussion addressing the challenges of diagnosing BPD when there is active AUD.

How to Make the Diagnoses

A collaborative approach can facilitate diagnostic clarification. Plain language descriptions of core criteria can be given to patients, and patients should have the opportunity to explain whether and why each criterion applies to them. In many cases, it is helpful to look together at the current DSM criteria and reflect on symptoms together, with the clinician explaining any technical language as needed. The diagnostic evaluation should also include an assessment of whether alcohol withdrawal management (detoxification) is needed (see Chapter 9, "Level-of-Care Considerations"), a safety assessment regarding potential for self-harm or other dangerous behaviors, and a determination of the need for medical evaluation of alcohol-related conditions such as liver inflammation (see Appendix E, "Screening Instruments").

In settings where interactions with patients are more time-limited, such as emergency departments or clinics, standardized screening tools may help make the diagnostic process efficient for the clinician and understandable for the patient. (See Appendix E for a full list of screening instruments.) Two such instruments are the McLean Screening Instrument for BPD (MSI-BPD; Zanarini et al. 2003) and the Alcohol Use Disorder Identification Test-Concise (AUDIT-C; Bush et al. 1998), which includes gender-based scoring (Table 4–2). Advantages of these tools are that they are self-reported questionnaires that are easy to administer and to score. One important caveat is that most screening instruments have had limited validation for people with both AUD and BPD. Patients will often benefit from having ample time to consider questions and their responses. It can also be helpful to review answers together in a collaborative fashion to clarify responses and provide normative feedback, such as typical drinking patterns among peers and health guidelines on alcohol consumption. For instance, adolescents and young adults may overestimate levels of drinking in their peer groups. Learning that their alcohol use exceeds that of most peers may motivate them to reduce their intake (Agostinelli et al. 1995).

It is important to remember that all screening tools will produce false-positive and false-negative results in some cases. Clinical judgment should always be used to finalize any diagnosis. Screening tools are best used as one component of a comprehensive assessment. (Please see Appendix E for a more complete listing of screening tools.)

When making a diagnosis, involvement of loved ones can be very helpful, if permitted by the patient. Family and friends provide useful collateral information to clarify diagnoses. This is also an opportune time to provide patient and family with education on diagnoses and what to expect from treatment (see later section, "Patient and Family Education"). Significant others (spouses, partners, boyfriends/girlfriends) can help by fostering a supportive environment that is conducive to achieving the treatment goals established for BPD and AUD. Their collaboration should be sought whenever possible.

Assessing Motivation to Make Changes

Patients enter treatment with varying levels of willingness to engage in behavioral change. At times, clinicians may anticipate one goal (such as cessation of alcohol use) while the patient has another in mind (such as improvement in mood). The transtheoretical model of behavioral change

Table 4–2. Screening instruments (see also Appendix E)

Name	Abbreviation	Format	Access	Reference
Borderline personality disorder				
McLean Screening Instrument for Borderline Personality Disorder	MSI-BPD	10 items, yes/no	A measure of DSM Section II criteria; available online (NovoPsych 2024)	Zanarini et al. 2003
Zanarini Rating Scale for Borderline Personality Disorder	ZAN-BPD	9 items, rated 0–4	Available online (Scribd 2024)	Zanarini et al. 2015
Borderline Symptom List 23	BSL-23	23 items, rated 0–4	See Appendix E; also available online (University of Washington 2024)	Bohus et al. 2009
Borderline Symptom List Behavior Supplement	BSL-SUPP	11 items, rated 0–4	See Appendix E; also available online (University of Washington 2024)	Bohus et al. 2009
Personality Assessment Inventory-Borderline	PAI-BOR	24 items, rated 0–3	Limited availability	Morey and Boggs 2004
Screening Instrument for Borderline Personality Disorder	PI-Bord	5 items, 4-point scale	Available online (APA 2024)	Lohanan et al. 2020
Five-Factor Borderline Inventory (self-report and informant versions)	FFBI	120 items, rated 1–5, with 12 subscales	Limited availability	Mullins-Sweatt et al. 2012; Min et al. 2021

Table 4–2. Screening instruments (see also Appendix E) *(continued)*

Name	Abbreviation	Format	Access	Reference
Alcohol use disorder				
Alcohol Use Disorders Identification Test	AUDIT	10 items, rated 0–4	Available online (National Institute on Drug Abuse 2024)	Bradley et al. 2003
Alcohol Use Disorders Identification Test-Concise	AUDIT-C	3 items, rated 0–4	See Appendix E; also available online (National Institute on Drug Abuse 2024)	Bradley et al. 2003
Alcohol Use Disorders Identification Test-Piccinelli Consumption	AUDIT-PC	5 items	Intended for primary care setting; see Appendix E	Piccinelli et al. 1997
Clinical Institute Withdrawal Assessment-Alcohol, Revised	CIWA-Ar	10 items, rated 1–7	See Appendix E	Sullivan et al. 1989
Short Alcohol Withdrawal Scale	SAWS	10 items, rated 0–3	See Appendix E	Gossop et al. 2002
Addiction Severity Index		Single question	See Appendix E	McLellan et al. 1992
American Society of Addiction Medicine Patient Placement Criteria	ASAM-PPC	9 levels and sublevels; 6 dimensions	See Appendix E	Hoffman 1993
Cut down, annoyed, guilty, eye-opener	CAGE	4 items, yes/no	See Appendix E; also available online (Johns Hopkins Medicine 2024)	Ewing 1984

can be a helpful framework for assessing and understanding readiness to change (Table 4–3). This model designates a stage of change (pre-contemplation, contemplation, preparation, action, and maintenance) based on the patient's motivation or readiness, which can then guide treatment interventions. For example, patients in the *contemplation* stage may be open to information such as normative feedback in actively evaluating their problem behavior (e.g., drinking alcohol) (Prochaska and DiClemente 1982). In contrast, clinicians may need to be gentle and cautious about offering information to those in the *pre-contemplation* stage, as by definition, they do not see their behavior as a problem (Krebs et al. 2018).

Clinically, the transtheoretical model has limitations. The process of change often moves in a nonlinear fashion and may cycle back and forth between levels of motivation. The demarcation between stages is not as discrete as the model would suggest. Whether or not a clinician decides to use the model in treatment, it is important to assess motivation and use empirically supported interventions such as motivational interviewing (MI) to elicit, explore, and resolve the patient's ambivalence to change.

A particular strength of the transtheoretical model lies in its synergy with MI. MI can be applied not only to drinking behavior, but also to other self-destructive behaviors (e.g., symptoms of BPD). The GPM clinician can begin to use an MI approach starting in the initial encounter (see "Motivational Interviewing" later in this chapter).

Assessment of Behavioral Precipitants and Reinforcers

For most patients with BPD+AUD, interpersonal stressors can be important precipitants that bring on symptoms or exacerbate them, including drinking episodes. Some interpersonal stressors can be thought of as "push factors" for drinking behaviors. These may be situations that create uncomfortable emotions that, in turn, push a person to use alcohol as a coping or avoidance strategy. Abusive or exploitative relationships, abandonment fears, interpersonal disappointments, and social isolation may function in this manner in patients with BPD. Likewise, other social factors, including seemingly positive or innocuous situations, may act as "pull factors" toward alcohol use as a means of producing or enhancing pleasurable emotions. For instance, a highly valued new relationship may pull a patient toward drinking, particularly when it involves a partner who uses alcohol. Alcohol is used habitually in dating and sexual activities, which can transform otherwise healthy interactions into potential triggers.

Table 4–3. Stages of change in the transtheoretical model

Pre-contemplative	Not recognizing that it would be beneficial to change a behavior because the behavior is not recognized as problematic
Contemplative	Recognizing at least some aspect of behavior as problematic, and thus willing to consider a change
Preparation	Determining that behavior change is important or necessary and therefore planning to make a change
Action	Taking intentional steps to change behavior
Maintenance	Sustaining behavioral change

Source. Prochaska and DiClemente 1982.

Given that maladaptive behaviors are central to the suffering caused by both AUD and BPD, basic techniques of behavioral analysis and contingency management are often very helpful. Through the process of classical conditioning, previously neutral stimuli that are repeatedly paired with precipitants for alcohol use or other reinforcing behaviors can come to independently produce a desire to engage in these behaviors. The 12-step program language of "people, places, and things" will be familiar to many people with even minimal exposure to the recovery community and may serve as an entry point to this discussion. Internal states such as fatigue or depression may make it harder to use skills and engage in adaptive behavior. Internal states may also become conditioned stimuli themselves, as long-standing behavior patterns produce learned associations with problematic behaviors. In this way, emotional distress may produce a desire to engage in nonsuicidal self-injury, and fatigue or even positive emotions may become associated with an urge to drink to relax or unwind.

The GPM model of self and relationship functioning (i.e., connected, threatened, alone, and despair states; see Figures 2–1 and 2–2) can also be useful in understanding the interplay of alcohol use and BPD. For instance, in the *connected* state, attempts to use alcohol to manage anxiety and facilitate social connection may backfire if alcohol-related behavior destabilizes relationships. In the *threatened* or *despair* state, alcohol use may disinhibit nonsuicidal self-injury or frank suicidal behavior, respectively. Like motivation, the current level of functioning may fluctuate, necessitating repeated assessments over the course of treatment.

From the outset of treatment, many patients will describe triggers that lead to symptom exacerbations. The term *trigger* is useful as common parlance that is generally acceptable to lay people; however, it should be noted that the term can imply a lack of agency on the part of patients. Irrespective of the patient's language or level of insight when describing these experiences, it remains important to explore details in a collaborative process that will deepen understanding, for both patient and clinician, of the pattern of symptoms and precipitants. Patients should be engaged in a systematic self-inventory of past triggers to uncover associations that may not be obvious to them. Exploring past symptom exacerbations or relapses is often a productive approach to help patients better understand environmental or internal triggers.

The model of operant conditioning describes the way in which contingent rewards or punishments may increase or decrease the likelihood of an unwanted behavior. For example, pleasant near-term effects of alcohol may reinforce further drinking episodes. In a similar fashion, self-injury or threatened suicide may inadvertently be reinforced by the resulting temporary increase in engagement of loved ones or clinicians. Long-term consequences of alcohol misuse, self-injury, or suicidal statements are indeed aversive, but immediate effects are neurobiologically much more salient in influencing future behaviors. Exploration of such contingent reinforcers should be both thorough and tactful, describing the consequent behavior as understandable and, in its way, functional. It is particularly important not to dismiss suicidal or self-injurious behaviors as mere "attention seeking," although some patients may describe their own behavior in such terms. People who engage in nonsuicidal self-injury are at increased risk of suicidal behaviors (Zlotnick et al. 1997). See Chapter 6, "Managing Suicidality and Nonsuicidal Self-Injury," for details on responding to self-harm and suicidal behaviors.

The discussion of contingent reinforcement can be presented as a means of putting patients in the driver's seat, enhancing agency by finding alternate, healthy means to achieve goals such as experiencing pleasant feelings and social support. Although it is an important component of a thorough evaluation, the assessment of contingencies best takes place after first establishing a therapeutic alliance.

Assessment of Individual Strengths and Severity of Symptoms

A diagnostic evaluation often focuses on symptoms and vulnerabilities, but it is essential not to overlook a patient's strengths and past successes as part of the initial assessment. A focus on strengths and capabilities can bolster self-esteem, which in turn enhances hopeful motivation. If a patient describes a period of remission, ask how they accomplished it. Specifically, inquire about useful coping strategies, life circumstances, involvement in treatment or mutual help, and work or interpersonal situations that may have been stabilizing factors. In the same way that an investigation into precipitants of a past relapse can be quite informative, patient and provider will learn useful strategies by exploring past periods of improved functioning.

In addition to the presence or absence of symptoms as criteria for specific diagnoses, the severity of symptoms can help guide treatment. Specialized addiction care may be most appropriate for those with more severe AUD (see Figure 4–1). This group of people may have the most difficulty curtailing or controlling drinking and related problems without intensive support. Often, abstinence is the most realistic and appropriate treatment goal for this group, although many patients will not initially share such a goal. Abstinence-based support groups such as Alcoholics Anonymous tend to be more readily accepted by those with more severe AUD (Krentzman et al. 2011). People with severe AUD may also be more likely to benefit from treatment with FDA-approved medicines to promote drinking reduction and sustained abstinence (e.g., naltrexone, acamprosate, and disulfiram; see Chapter 7, "Pharmacotherapy for Co-occurring BPD and AUD"). Clinical trials of these medications generally involved subjects with more severe forms of AUD (Burnette et al. 2022).

Although many patients will experience improvement or at least stabilization of BPD symptoms during periods of abstinence from alcohol, some may experience a paradoxical flare-up of symptoms due to the absence of alcohol use as a coping mechanism for difficult feelings or unhealthy relationship dynamics. This pattern is important to recognize and acknowledge with patients, because the short-term relief that alcohol provides may be particularly reinforcing for people with this experience. Over time, many can gain a long-term perspective about the detrimental effects of alcohol on the trajectory of BPD symptoms and their lives overall.

Patient and Family Education

After making the diagnoses, the next important step is psychoeducation with the patient, as well as loved ones when appropriate. For people who may have been told their illness is the result of personal weakness or moral failure, education on the heritability and overlapping neurobiol-

Table 4–4. Key facts in disclosing the diagnoses

BPD and AUD commonly co-occur	BPD is more common among people with AUD AUD is more common among people with BPD
Co-occurrence of AUD and BPD may lead to greater severity of both disorders	Alcohol use may increase BPD symptoms, including unstable relationships and sense of self, impulsivity, anger outbursts, and risk of self-harm Active BPD symptoms may precipitate attempts to self-medicate with alcohol and may make it more difficult to control impulses to drink
AUD and BPD both need evidence-based treatment for optimal outcomes	Presence of an SUD makes remission of BPD less likely Co-occurrence of BPD and an SUD increases suicide risk beyond either disorder alone Co-occurrence of BPD and an SUD is associated with greater social and psychological dysfunction and a more persistent course of both disorders
AUD and BPD can be successfully treated— remission is possible	In long-term studies of people with BPD, remission rates for both BPD and SUDs are high (85%–90%) Relapse rates are lower with sustained remission
BPD and AUD are both heritable illnesses	At the population level, ~50% of the variability in AUD and ~42% of the variability in BPD are due to genetic factors
BPD and AUD may share common neurobiological pathways	Brain pathways associated with emotional drives (fight, flight, reward) are relatively overactive, while those associated with cognitive control are relatively underactive
BPD and AUD both respond to stress	Both benefit from supportive, predictably structured environments

Note. AUD = alcohol use disorder; BPD = borderline personality disorder; SUD = substance use disorder.
Source. Distel et al. 2008; Gunderson and Links 2014; McGirr et al. 2007; Tomko et al. 2014; Verhulst et al. 2015; Zanarini et al. 2011a

ogy of BPD and AUD can validate their experiences and reduce stigma (Table 4–4). Medicalizing both disorders creates an objective and nonjudgmental framework, signaling that treatment aims to reduce symptoms and enhance functioning. An optimistic approach can motivate patients to anticipate positive aspects of recovery while communicating the importance of ongoing treatment to achieve and sustain goals. Following is a sample script on how to communicate the diagnoses and basic education about them:

> BPD and AUD are common diagnoses that often co-occur. They are both heritable disorders that share neurobiological pathways, meaning that the disorders run in families and may have overlapping neurobiological causes. Individuals with BPD are predisposed to being highly interpersonally sensitive, which leads to unstable relationships as well as intense emotional reactions and impulsive behavior when feeling rejected or slighted. They also may experience a sense of shame about feeling inherently bad. Individuals with AUD are highly sensitive to the effects of alcohol, which may lead to difficulty controlling their drinking behavior. Often individuals with BPD and co-occurring AUD may use alcohol to cope with their intense negative emotions, leading to further loss of control and self-destructive impulsive behavior. BPD and AUD each intensify the symptoms of the other. The good news is that both BPD and AUD are treatable, and there are good outcomes when both disorders are appropriately addressed. (adapted from Gunderson and Links 2014, pp. 23–24)

As outlined in Chapter 2, "Overall Principles," providing education about diagnoses is a core therapeutic procedure of GPM-AUD. Providing diagnostic labels without context can lead anxious patients and family members to seek other sources of information. An uncurated search of the internet by a newly diagnosed patient or loved one will likely produce misleading anecdotes, myths, stigmatizing commentary, and misconceptions. Conversely, engaging patients and families in psychoeducation can set realistic, hopeful expectations for treatment and recovery. It is also important to be frank about the limits of current knowledge on best practices. Humility about what is not known will help keep expectations reasonable while modeling "good-enough" aspects of relationship dynamics that are also central to GPM-AUD.

Motivational Interviewing

For clients who have subthreshold or mild AUD, or for those who have not accepted the diagnosis (see next section, "Common Problems"), MI may be an especially useful intervention (Table 4–5). This approach to working with patients on a range of behavioral health issues was influenced by the person-centered stance of Carl Rogers (Goldfried 2007) and the transtheoretical model of behavioral change described earlier in this chapter (Prochaska and DiClemente 1982). MI includes a set of principles that keeps the patient perspective at the forefront, while facilitating discussion of ambivalence about substance use and reasons to make healthy changes. Use of MI can help avoid unnecessary conflict and foster nonjudgmental self-exploration.

Clinical trials have supported brief MI as an effective intervention for mild alcohol-related problems, in addition to diagnosed AUD (Vasilaki et al. 2006). MI can be useful for many patient populations and across different diagnoses and behavioral targets (Bischof et al. 2021). Further, MI can start when clients are in the pre-contemplative or contemplative stage of change, and key elements of the intervention are aimed at promoting readiness to change (Miller 1983). Research supports change-promotion techniques in MI (e.g., reflective listening and amplifying *change talk*—that is, any statements favoring behavior change) as mechanisms of change in treatment (Apodaca and Longabaugh 2009). MI techniques such as these are behaviorally focused and do not require the client to accept their diagnosis or for the symptoms to be severe to move forward with them. MI's orientation, spirit, and change-promotion techniques make it a suitable starting point for clients along the entire spectrum of alcohol-related problems. Fundamental techniques of MI are described in Table 4–5. General information on MI, including information on how to pursue training in this approach, can be found online (e.g., Motivational Interviewing Network of Trainers 2024).

MI and GPM share a stance of curiosity and uncertainty, encouraging autonomy, accountability, and self-exploration. MI is consistently client-centered, with a focus on open-ended questions, validation, clarification, and drawing out each patient's individual values and goals. However, practitioners of MI do not simply listen and reflect back to patients in a neutral fashion. *Change talk* is elicited and reinforced while acknowledg-

Table 4-5.   Core principles and techniques of motivational interviewing

Spirit

Nonjudgmental
Positive regard
Curious

Skills

Evocation	Ask open-ended questions.
	Over- or understate the patient's perspective to push them to hold the other side.
	Explore pros and cons of drinking.
	Discuss goals and values.
Affirmations	Find opportunities to genuinely and naturally express how you value and appreciate the client.
Reflections	Simple: repeat what the client said.
	Deeper: repeat the meaning you sensed.
	On feelings: focus on the emotional content.

Strategy

Engaging	When the client engages in change talk, encourage them to elaborate.
Focusing	Allow exploration when time allows, and gently bring the client back to the topic of their drinking and BPD symptoms when needed.
Evoking	Avoid confrontational interactions with your client by maintaining the spirit of MI, while using evocation techniques to encourage change talk.
Planning	In addition to general hopes, identify some specific, attainable goals. Help the client form an action plan to meet their goals.

Note.   BPD = borderline personality disorder; MI = motivational interviewing.
Source.   Data from Miller and Rollnick 2023.

ing patient ambivalence. The process of establishing treatment expectations at the onset of treatment can be consistent with MI if it is client-centered and collaborative. Clinical opinions, recommendations, and even advice can be consistent with MI. Such feedback should be given after asking permission and should be accompanied by repeatedly soliciting patient input.

Common Problems

It Is Unclear Whether Symptoms Are Due to BPD, AUD, or Both

Some patients may present in settings primarily focused on the treatment of BPD. Others may present for AUD, and BPD symptoms become evident during the course of evaluation and treatment. Still others may identify insomnia, anxiety, depression, relationship difficulties, or other problems as primary treatment priorities. The simultaneous presence of multiple symptoms across different domains can make diagnostic assessment complex and challenging.

Several approaches can help clarify a diagnosis of BPD in people who drink heavily. Often, typical symptoms of BPD will persist (although possibly improve) during periods of extended abstinence. For some people, BPD symptoms may be present before the onset of regular alcohol use or the development of AUD. A careful history and consideration of information from collateral sources can be helpful.

Diagnosis of AUD when a patient has a presentation suggestive of BPD also presents a challenge in part because impulsive substance use is itself a criterion for BPD. It may be most challenging to delineate mild AUD from the impulsive, risky alcohol use that is a common symptom of BPD. A practical approach may be taken in managing such problematic alcohol use, starting with less intensive treatment. This might start with a functional assessment of the patient's alcohol use, followed by an MI approach to 1) identify where and how alcohol use is causing or exacerbating problems in the patient's life; 2) set goals for appropriate alcohol use (this may mean abstinence); and 3) plan specific strategies and steps toward achieving those goals. Treatment intensity can then be increased if improvement is not apparent.

The overlap between criteria for BPD and for mild AUD raises the question of whether BPD is overdiagnosed in those who have substance use disorders. In one study of co-occurring BPD and substance use disorders, when substance use was excluded as a possible criterion for BPD, 23% no longer met criteria for BPD (Dulit et al. 1990). Thus the majority will continue to meet criteria; for others, borderline symptoms will remain important as a focus of treatment even if the impulsivity criterion is no longer met.

The Patient Does Not Agree With the Diagnoses

Some patients experience certain terms as stigmatizing. Although many individuals in recovery from substance use disorders self-identify as "alcoholics" or "addicts," other patients find these terms pejorative. It is best for clinicians to use DSM-5-TR or ICD-11 terminology. It is also important to use language that does not identify a person as their diagnosis (for instance, say "person with alcohol use disorder" rather than "alcohol abuser"; say "a person with borderline personality disorder" rather than "a borderline"). If the patient rejects the diagnoses outright, it may be more practical to agree on a set of problems, symptoms, and goals as a focus for treatment. Patients may prefer to use terms such as *harmful alcohol use, impaired emotion regulation,* or *interpersonal hypersensitivity problems.* The set of techniques described earlier for MI may be particularly helpful for patients who are unsure about diagnoses of AUD or BPD and for those who are ambivalent about changing maladaptive behavior.

Conclusion

Diagnosing and providing patient education about co-occurring AUD and BPD can be a therapeutic intervention in itself. By providing an opportunity for goal setting, normative feedback, and motivational enhancement strategies, diagnosis begins the process of productive clinical engagement. By identifying the inherent vulnerabilities of AUD and BPD (i.e., impulsivity, deficits in self-protection, and in the case of BPD, high levels of interpersonal sensitivity), the clinician can enhance patient agency and guide helpful self-management strategies.

Assessment may best be viewed as a continuous process, starting with the diagnostic interview during initial meetings and continuing with ongoing assessment of symptoms, self and relational states, maladaptive or recovery-oriented behaviors, and environmental and intrapersonal precipitants. Through a collaborative process, clinician, patient, and loved ones can map a course toward relief from symptoms and full enjoyment of healthy, meaningful life activities.

5

Setting the Framework

Daniel Price, M.D.
Erik Ydrefelt, M.Sc. Psych

Good psychiatric management (GPM) starts with the pragmatic attitude that effectiveness should drive treatment. Although this manual spells out a structure to GPM of borderline personality disorder (BPD) and alcohol use disorder (AUD), clinicians should use their own good judgment to develop a treatment first and foremost that is useful to the individual (personalized treatment). This attitude will guide decisions about, for example, the frequency of sessions and the duration of treatment. As they progress, clinicians will learn to emphasize this pragmatic approach based on observable results, while also enlisting the patient (and relevant family members) in monitoring whether progress is being made in terms of goals jointly formulated at the outset.

GPM fosters an expectation of change and emphasizes the responsibility of the patient to build a stable and meaningful life outside of treatment. Accountability, flexibility, thoughtfulness, and an active (not reactive) stance are all basic principles of GPM-AUD, as discussed in Chapter 2. Following is a sample clinician statement proposing a therapy relationship that is real as well as professional; indeed, this serves as early psychoeducation about how treatment will go, and how it will be assessed:

> We will start by meeting weekly, but how often and how long we meet will depend on whether our time together is useful. As with drinking, more is not always better. We will be able to judge whether the treatment is helpful by paying attention to whether you feel better and whether your problem drinking, impulsivity, self-harm, and relationship difficulties improve over time. I will need your help, and the help of those most involved in your life, to frequently assess this. Is that something you are willing to do with me?

Treatment usually begins with weekly sessions. More frequent sessions may not be possible in high-volume clinical settings with lower staff or because of the patient's schedule. Higher frequency is advisable only if the patient is using the sessions to reach goals, and even then, two sessions per week is the maximum advisable frequency for individual counseling. Adjunctive counseling—such as substance group therapies, mutual-support coaching, and vocational counseling for finances, housing, and employment—may be appropriate for patients in early recovery. Prototypically, those with BPD idealize dependencies, so according to the GPM-AUD approach, treatment should not occupy too much space in the week at the expense of other life-building activities (Table 5–1). Split treatments and more peer-oriented work in groups and mutual-help communities (see Chapter 8, "Multimodal Treatments") will mitigate dependence and extend the patient's social network, providing a holding environment to counteract the intolerance of aloneness that drives BPD symptoms, as well as reliance on alcohol to manage stress.

Primary GPM-AUD clinicians are often not psychiatrists, so medication management by a collaborating prescribing professional (e.g., primary care provider, nurse practitioner, physician assistant) may be indicated at particular junctures of treatment (see Chapter 7, "Pharmacotherapy for Co-occurring BPD and AUD"). The patient should be informed that, when they work with another clinician for medications or group treatment, the clinicians together form a care team, and release of information between care team members is necessary to achieve optimal outcomes. For this patient population, medications are indicated for the

Table 5-1.   GPM-AUD framework

- Sessions are held once a week, twice a week if indicated and helpful.
- Duration depends on progress (but expect 12–18 months for initial stabilization).
- Adjunctive treatments (peer support, group therapy, family education, medications) are useful; care team collaboration is important for good outcomes.
- Consultation and peer discussions are encouraged as a practice of good clinical management.

Note.   GPM-AUD = good psychiatric management for borderline personality disorder and alcohol use disorder.
Source.   Adapted from Gunderson and Links 2014.

management of alcohol use problems or other co-occurring disorders as is standard of care, but there is no medication specifically approved by the FDA for treatment of BPD.

The treatment of BPD+AUD can be challenging to contain, conceptualize, and organize. Consultation with other clinicians allows the treating clinician to take stock and develop a coherent narrative of the problems at hand (see Table 5–1). Regular peer discussions provide a predictable and nonreactive forum for maintaining perspective. Consultation also extends the social network of the treatment process itself, rather than limiting treatment to an exclusive intense relationship to which the patient is hypersensitive and dependent. Special in-depth consultations may be necessary if progress is not as expected or has stalled (see next section, "Assessing Progress").

GPM-AUD uses resources that already exist and are naturally available in one's clinical environment, rather than requiring clinicians to develop specialized resources that are difficult to start up or maintain (see Appendix D). Most patients will benefit from another form of treatment, particularly mutual-help groups such as Alcoholics Anonymous (AA), Narcotics Anonymous, or SMART Recovery (Fein and Nip 2012). These interventions are free and available virtually around the clock. More formal, clinician-led groups (e.g., skills groups, interpersonal groups) can be helpful, although their effectiveness should be assessed regularly (see Chapter 8, "Multimodal Treatments").

Family involvement should be discussed with the patient early in treatment. When the patient is financially dependent on or living with parents, clinician contact with the family is strongly encouraged. Patients might be reluctant, but better understanding of the process may make their loved ones more helpful and supportive, a point that should get patients on board. To set the frame around family involvement, the clinician needs to clarify that they will not be offering family therapy. Instead, they will focus on providing psychoeducation, planning, solving problems, assessing progress, and identifying resources (see Chapter 8, "Multimodal Treatment," and Appendix C).

Assessing Progress

Working as a group to monitor change and progress highlights different points of view and demonstrates to the patient the investment their team and their loved ones have made in their recovery. The patient should experience an improvement in subjective distress, behavior, interpersonal relating, and social functioning (Table 5–2), but change is not a linear process, especially with BPD+AUD. The more severe the illness, the more likely are relapse and remission. When change fails to occur, it is important to recognize it, identify and address hindrances, and make sure the diagnostic formulation has not overlooked other treatable conditions, such as trauma- and stressor-related disorders, ADHD, or other substance use disorders (SUDs), all of which are highly prevalent in the BPD+AUD population.

It is imperative that clinicians monitor their own worries or negative thoughts about treatment progress to prevent burnout and optimize good clinical outcomes. If the answers to the questions in Table 5–3 are "no," then the clinician should consult with colleagues and reassess the patient's diagnosis and treatment structure.

The clinician can also ask about the patient's progress in terms of essential factors that enable patients to process emotions, make meaning of their experience, and improve their self-esteem enough to sustain the challenges of change. The questions in Table 5–4 are appropriate at various stages of treatment.

Getting started in GPM involves setting goals to assess treatment effectiveness. To make this a fundamental way of evaluating the treatment in the early stages, raise the question explicitly. Staking the treatment's value in effectiveness (rather than the oscillations of the rescue/rejection dynamic inherent to both BPD and AUD interpersonal dynamics) helps stabilize the predictable challenges to the therapeutic alliance. Table 5–5 lists reasons to question the treatment at particular stages. The clinician should actively monitor the treatment, and if the patient does not show

Table 5–2. Expected changes

Target area	Change expected	Time	Interventions
Subjective distress	↓ Anxiety and depression or dysphoria ↓ Cravings if engaged in abstinence plan (2–3 months) or drinking reduction plan (6 months or longer)	2–3 months	↑ Support, situational change ↑ Self-awareness
Behavior	↓ Alcohol use, self-harm, promiscuity, suicidality, rages	2–6 months	↑ Awareness of self and interpersonal triggers, problem-solving strategies, utilizing recovery network
Interpersonal	↑ Empathy toward self/other ↑ Assertiveness (proportionate to circumstances) ↓ Devaluation and idealization ↓ Neediness ↑ Healthy collaboration with therapist and others	6–12 months	↑ Mentalizing, stability of attachment, grieving loss of idealized parents
Social function	↑ School/work/home responsibilities and relationships ↓ Identification with therapist ↑ Differentiation from therapist	12–18 months	↑ Grieving loss of idealized therapist

Source. Adapted from Gunderson and Links 2014.

Table 5-3.   Clinician thoughts and experiences to monitor

- Do I understand my patient better?
- Can I predict my patient's reactions? (What triggers alcohol relapse, anger, self-harm, suicidality?)
- Do I find myself increasingly connected? (Do I think about the patient between sessions?)
- Does the patient trust me as being well-intentioned? Does the patient collaborate with me?
- Is the patient able to bring up areas of disagreement during sessions?

Source.   Adapted from Gunderson and Links 2014.

Table 5-4.   Patient thoughts and experiences to monitor and discuss

- Does the patient feel safe here? Does the patient experience you as being supportive of independent decision-making and able to maintain appropriate boundaries?
- Have your patient's anger, guilt, and self-destructiveness decreased as they wrestle with the question of whether they have a right to be angry?
- Does your patient believe in their personal value, that they are worthwhile?
- Is your patient preparing for the end of treatment?

Source.   Data from Gregory 2022.

expected signs of improvement, then the clinician should consider consultation.

Intersession Availability

The emotional instability and interpersonal hypersensitivity of patients with BPD+AUD frequently lead to crises. Intersession availability (whether and how the patient can reach out to the clinician or services for support between scheduled sessions) is a crucial part of the treatment frame. For BPD, there has been little consensus on what constitutes optimal availability. Among the evidence-based treatments, some see 24-hour as-needed intersession support as a key element; others explicitly try to minimize contact outside of scheduled appointments (Choi-Kain et al. 2016). The same is true in BPD with co-occurring AUD or SUDs: treatments with both high and low intersession availability have had promising results (Kienast et al. 2014).

Table 5–5. When to question whether treatment is failing

Time in treatment		Observation
Shorter term	Weeks	• Attendance is poor. • Subjective distress is not better. • Patient is not demonstrating any perceptible change in thought or behavior. • You do not like the patient.
	Months	• Substance use or self-injurious behaviors worsen. • Patient consistently disparages the therapy. • Your empathy or understanding of the patient has not improved.
Longer term	About 6 months	• Substance use or self-injurious behaviors persist. • Patient does not remember or use lessons from prior sessions. • Patient has not increased engagement in school or work activities. • Patient does not express a sense that they can feel safe in treatment. • Patient does not recognize significance of adverse interpersonal events such as rejection or separation. • Patient's ability to verbalize and tolerate painful unprocessed underlying emotions (such as anger or shame) is not improving.

Source. Adapted from Gunderson and Links 2014.

Availability of support between sessions relates to the patient's primary vulnerability and also their safety. Consistent with the GPM-AUD approach, 1) the parameters and rationale of intersession availability should be addressed early as part of the treatment framework; 2) intersession contact should occur only briefly and purposefully; 3) contact between clinican and patient should be maintained in a standard way even in times of crisis; and 4) any intersession contact should be assessed for whether it helps the patient achieve increased self-reliance (Jacob 2016).

Previous GPM tools have suggested that the clinician tell the patient to contact them if needed, without specifying in advance what "needed" means (Gunderson and Links 2014). This approach is not always feasible, and of the many ways for a patient to make contact (phone call, text, email, patient portal, etc.), not all are permitted by every clinician's system of care. Some are useful for appointment changes, conveying homework, or completing forms, and others are more appropriate for urgent matters. Beginning with what the clinician is able to offer (in the constraints of their system of practice and their own comfort), the clinician and patient can work collaboratively to agree on parameters of communication methods, frequency, and expectations (e.g., anticipated response time) (Figure 5–1). When patient and caregiver do interact between sessions, these contacts should be kept brief and purposeful, be documented in the clinical care record, and be reviewed in subsequent sessions. Clinicians must be explicit that no intersession contact with an intoxicated patient is appropriate. If intoxication is dangerous for any reason, patients can refer to their relapse plan and follow that algorithm (see Chapter 9, "Level-of-Care Considerations").

Regardless of the availability a clinician can offer patients, GPM emphasizes that the patient is responsible for managing their own safety between sessions. This responsibility does not necessarily mean managing crises alone, but it does mean utilizing an increasingly broader social network. In the case of GPM+AUD, patients should be reminded of the broader community that is available to them between sessions—including mutual-support meetings available virtually (e.g., In the Rooms), AA sponsors (with their agreement), and crisis counselors available through the 988 crisis line (see Chapter 6, "Managing Suicidality and Nonsuicidal Self-Injury").

When the relationship between patient and clinician is both professional and real, we can assume that intersession availability will carry significant emotional and interpersonal implications. Anticipate that patients may have difficulty adhering to the agreement, making it necessary to revisit whether intersession availability is helpful. Broadly, two scenarios necessitate this: overuse and underuse of availability.

Overuse of Availability

Some patients will reach out too frequently, and in situations they might manage independently. Use these situations to help the patient reflect on how they relate to their core issues, such as difficulties with being alone, fears that no one cares about them, and the like. By applying GPM prin-

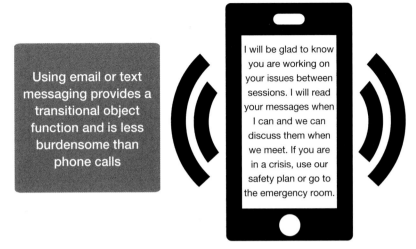

Figure 5–1. Intersession contact.

Intersession contacts should be kept brief and purposeful, be documented in the clinical
  care record, and be reviewed in subsequent sessions; no intersession contact with an intoxicated patient is appropriate.

ciples, clinicians can use these moments of perceived helplessness to foster patient agency and address dichotomous thinking. Inquire whether the patient feels that these calls are helpful, and if so, in what way. Encourage exploring other ways the situation might be managed.

Underuse of Availability

Conversely, a patient might avoid making contact, even during a crisis. As with the issue of overuse, address these situations to increase self-knowledge. Ask the patient why they did not try to reach out. Do they view the clinician as uncaring? Are they worried about overburdening the clinician? Might other interpersonal dynamics be at play?

In both scenarios, the clinician should approach the situation with a nonjudgmental attitude fostering curiosity. Deviations from the agreement offer opportunities to explore the interpersonal dynamics driving these behaviors and collaboratively find ways to navigate them, with the joint goal of increasing the patient's self-reliance.

Building Alliance

Creating a helpful working relationship with BPD patients can seem challenging at times. Given the interpersonal nature of their problems, that same relationship is also one of the main vehicles for change. In

**Table 5–6.	Sequential forms of therapeutic alliance**

Form of alliance	Description
Contractual (goals/roles)	Contractual alliance refers to setting the framework (schedule, fee, confidentiality) and establishing an agreement between patient and therapist on treatment goals and their roles in achieving them. Relevant to all modalities and can be established in the first session, but may take two or three sessions.
Relational (affective/ empathic)	Relational alliance refers to a therapist's perception of the patient as likable and understandable and to the patient's experience of the therapist as caring, understanding, and genuine. Can develop very quickly and should have developed by 6 months. If sustained, it is a corrective experience.
Working (cognitive/ motivational)	In a working alliance, the patient is a reliable collaborator who can recognize unwanted pain-inducing observations by a therapist as being well intended. Grows gradually, is especially relevant to individual psychotherapies, varies within sessions, and is unlikely to be reliably present in the first year.

Source.	Adapted from Gunderson and Links 2014.

GPM, a basic therapeutic stance of concerned attention, active listening, and continuous validation of the patient's experiences is the foundation on which the alliance is built (Table 5–6). The clinician must be able to meet some of the patient's needs for support and care and at the same time enable their autonomy and agency. And again, the therapy is a judgment-free zone (see the first principle of integrating dynamic deconstructive psychotherapy (DDP) into GPM, Chapter 3). It is important to note that for a BPD patient, it is an achievement (rather than a precondition) to trust the clinician's good intentions.

Besides the basic therapeutic stance, the following interventions usually facilitate alliance-building, as they serve to engage the patient in collaboration.

Psychoeducation

Psychoeducation serves several important functions, as noted in Chapter 4, "Making the Diagnoses." Besides instilling realistic hope, reducing shame, and serving to normalize medical illness, psychoeducation teaches the patient about self-assessment and evidence-based care strategies. Psychoeducation also gives the patient a chance to understand what is expected of them to make the treatment effective. To foster agency, the clinician should encourage the patient to also actively learn more about their disorders from reliable sources (e.g., Substance Abuse and Mental Health Services Administration [SAMHSA]) (see Appendix D).

Given the stigma surrounding both BPD and AUD, and that BPD patients are prone to experiencing destabilizing and painful shame, it is important to establish a medical framework. This can be done in several ways. An overview of the neurobiology that underlies BPD can be helpful, since it also illustrates how therapy works.

Again to foster agency, psychoeducation is an opportunity to discuss AUD and SUDs (see the third principle in integrating DDP and GPM, Chapter 3). The patient should learn how BPD and AUD symptoms can interact—that is, how both intoxication and hangover can worsen BPD symptoms. The following discussion is a way to see whether this makes sense to them:

> From what you are saying, it seems that the drinking helps you feel better in the moment when you're under a lot of stress. You are in the driver's seat to make an informed choice as to whether to continue it. What do you think about that? On the one hand, alcohol helps take the edge off of stressful situations, but on the other it is easy to lose control over the amount of alcohol you drink in a stress episode. One of the negative aspects of drinking is that it has a prolonged withdrawal syndrome that often worsens symptoms of borderline personality disorder for 1 to 2 days after drinking even relatively modest amounts. (Gregory 2022, p. 92)

Homework

The basic stance of GPM is that the patient needs to take responsibility for their recovery. One important way of doing so is finding ways to work on their self-understanding; in other words, they may practice connecting with their emotions and experiences between sessions. This should be part of psychoeducation. Some form of homework is encouraged, although this can take many forms. Some suggestions are shown in Table 5–7.

Setting Goals

Setting goals is an important part of treatment. Besides the overarching goals of the treatment, the patient should be encouraged to formulate short-term, feasible goals to work toward (Table 5–8). To facilitate agency, allow the patient to formulate what they would like to get out of treatment (Gregory 2019). With many patients, however, this is easier said than done—formulating goals that feel personally relevant and realistic can itself be a goal. Given the importance of staying in treatment (or returning if treatment is disrupted), that is one explicit goal.

Different Forms of Therapeutic Alliance

The therapeutic alliance builds on a multilayer foundation. GPM outlines three types of alliance on which clinician and patient can collaboratively build—the stability of one firms up the strength of the next.

Contractual Alliance

A contractual alliance refers to the basic framework and agreement between patient and clinician—basically, establishing goals and agreeing on what the clinician and the patient need to do to achieve them. This type of alliance is relevant to all modalities (e.g., medication management, psychotherapy, case management). It can usually be established in the first couple of sessions. Naturally, the agreement needs to be individualized so that it is relevant to the patient. And again, given the importance of remaining in treatment, the contract should be tailored to promote the patient's continuing participation in treatment.

Relational Alliance

A relational alliance refers to the patient's experience of the clinician as caring, understanding, and genuine, and to the clinician's perception of the patient as likable and understandable. This form of alliance can develop quickly or take some time, but it should generally have been established by 6 months. As a corrective experience, it is an important vehicle of change.

Table 5–7. Intersession homework

Form of homework	Rationale
Write an autobiography	Helps the patient to build a more coherent narrative, although some may find it difficult. Start simple by asking them to make a life chart with major events or a family tree. This foundation can then be enlarged and the details filled in as the treatment progresses.
Detail a recent crisis	Helps make sense of the events and feelings that drive self-destructive actions or dysregulation. A chain analysis or a mentalizing exploration of a recent crisis is a good (sometimes challenging) way to practice the higher-level emotional processing needed to build stability of this capacity under stress (see "Building Narratives," the second principle of integrating DDP and GPM in Chapter 3). The simple act of labeling emotions often soothes via top-down regulation in emotional processing.
Fill out structured forms	Self-assessments help the patient be involved in treatment between sessions and are easily adapted to varying treatment goals. The patient charts target symptoms to assess medication response (see Chapter 7, "Pharmacotherapy for Co-occurring BPD and AUD") or fills in safety plans. Regular self-assessment is a way of being aware of and labeling feelings. Keeping a daily drinking diary is a simple way for patient and clinician to accurately monitor the drinking reduction progress and how drinking episodes associate with BPD symptom severity.

Source. Data from Gunderson and Links 2014.

Table 5–8. Other interventions to supplement goal-setting

• Active but nonjudgmental exploration when patients are having difficulties with meeting treatment expectations.

• Coaching about situations (without overtaking the patient's autonomy or trying to resolve their ambivalence for them).

• In some cases, helping patients do what they feel unable to do for themselves (e.g., help set up appointments).

• Check in routinely regarding drinking behavior.

Source. Data from Gunderson and Links 2014.

Working Alliance

When a working alliance is established, the patient becomes a reliable collaborator. One important sign of this is that the patient is capable of using the clinician's observations, even when they might be painful to consider. The patient will also be able to consider the clinician as a real person (as opposed to an idealized or devalued one), as a result of gradual improvement in differentiating between self and other. This form of alliance takes time and grows gradually; it can also change within a session. It is not reliably present in the first year of treatment.

Common Problems

Changing Therapists

One of the guiding principles of GPM is that change is expected. If treatment with a therapist is ineffective or harmful, as evidenced by a lack of improvement or worsening of symptoms in crucial areas of safety (e.g., self-harm, suicide attempts, hospitalizations, or drinking behavior, with employment or legal consequences), then a change may be warranted. Problems arise when the patient or current therapist disagrees with the recommendation (for example, the therapist may see the recommendation as an attack on their competence). Therefore, it is important to depersonalize the recommendation for a change in treater by focusing on a lack of improvement in symptoms; emphasize that a change in treaters is not uncommon. If the patient is resistant to a change in therapist, then consider follow-up in several months or resuming care with that therapist once the crucial problem behaviors have changed.

Patient Refuses to Accept the Framework

A practical treatment framework is one that has some degree of flexibility, but the treatment is significantly handicapped if the patient refuses essential components, such as granting permission to confer or collaborate with other clinicians or family members, defining goals, addressing drinking (see section "Motivational Interviewing" in Chapter 4), or seeking help when suicidal. It is possible that as a therapeutic alliance develops through a real-and-professional relationship, the degree of resistance may decrease. Only when you have concluded that the resistance is incompatible with the patient's safety or with your ability to be helpful should treatment be suspended. Other factors that are incompatible with treatment include nonpayment, missing appointments, or refusal to adopt any reasonable safety plan.

Patient Is Not Able to Relate or Feel Connected to Treater

Effective treatment requires a connection between the patient and treater, so a lack of connection can be a problem when initiating treatment. It may take some time for a patient with BPD+AUD to form a stable attachment. If the disconnection is a form of dissociation, then the patient may benefit from psychoeducation or grounding exercises. If the lack of connection persists for eight or more appointments, then the treater should pursue a referral, help the patient find someone they might connect with, and also be ready for the patient to return.

You Don't Like Your Patient

It is important to acknowledge that dislike of a patient will interfere with treatment efficacy. If the reasons for dislike are universal (e.g., hygiene, dismissiveness, disrespect, or silence), this should be discussed, and the patient should be given an opportunity to change. If the dislike is a result of your personal aversions (e.g., appearance, politics, dependence, hostility), these (as countertransference issues) should be discussed with a consultant or peer to clarify what internal experiences are contributing. If they are beyond your ability to change, consider—with due apologies— telling the patient that you consider yourself a bad match because of your own limitations and that they deserve to work with someone more apt to be compatible. Not every clinician is a good fit for every patient. Understanding the source of the mismatch is the most constructive starting point to address it.

You Will Be Unavailable for an Extended Time

Occasionally, the treater will be unavailable for an extended period of time. As much as possible, the patient should be responsible for planning any treatment contacts. If plans allow, it may be reasonable for the treater to be available by email, phone, or online. A covering provider should be available as well. It is important for the clinician to recognize that periods away can be difficult for the patient (the patient may experience feelings of anger, rejection, or betrayal), and the patient should be encouraged to discuss this in treatment (before and after the absence).

Conclusion

GPM uses a pragmatic framework that enlists the patient and family in monitoring progress toward jointly formulated goals, alongside the clinician. Change is to be expected, so it is important to actively assess subjective distress, problematic behavior, and interpersonal and social function. If the patient is not progressing in these areas, consultation should be sought. Factors such as interpersonal hypersensitivity can make intersession availability both tricky and a powerful basis for change. The clinician-patient relationship is both professional and real, and collaborative agreement on parameters of intersession availability is crucial. Intersession contact should be brief, consistent (even in crisis), and continually assessed for whether it is promoting or discouraging long-term self-reliance.

Psychoeducation, homework, and goal setting can strengthen the patient-clinician alliance. In particular, psychoeducation about BPD and AUD—emphasizing the medical framework—can reduce stigma and shame, instill hope, and foster agency. Homework can amplify these salutary aspects of psychoeducation. Setting overarching goals as well as more short-term, achievable goals enhances patient agency, and the collaborative process can increase alliance. Progressive change in alliance is expected, from the concrete *contractual* alliance, through the increasingly interdependent *relational* alliance, to the realistic *working* alliance. The development of the alliance, like all expected change, should be jointly monitored by patient and clinician, and if it is not progressing as expected, consultation or a change in treatment should be considered.

6

Managing Suicidality and Nonsuicidal Self-Injury

Marcos S. Croci, M.D.
Robert J. Gregory, M.D.
Kimberley Siscoe, M.D.
Marcelo J. A. A. Brañas, M.D.
Lois W. Choi-Kain, M.D., M.Ed.

Suicidality is a leading concern in borderline personality disorder (BPD), and many clinicians are fearful of managing BPD patients because of the realistic risk of the patient's death by suicide. In alcohol use disorder (AUD) as well as BPD, the main acute causes of death are suicide (defined as self-injury with intention to die) and recklessly impulsive behaviors that place the person at risk for fatal injury. Although less dangerous in the immediate term, nonsuicidal self-injury (NSSI), which includes banging the head or cutting, punching, or burning parts of the body, is a major risk factor for suicide (Kapur et al. 2013), and the two are best understood as different levels of severity on a shared spectrum of psychopathology. Any effective treatment applied to self-injuring or self-destructive patients has to incorporate a procedure for managing safety, and interventions must be tailored to the clinical situation at hand (Brañas et al. 2022).

Historically, BPD has been associated with self-harm and suicide. Although NSSI is not specific to BPD, 90% of patients with BPD report self-harm (Goodman et al. 2017); thus self-harm is a signal to include BPD in the differential diagnosis (Reichl and Kaess 2021). Three-quarters of BPD patients attempt suicide (Black et al. 2004), and ~6% die by suicide (Temes et al. 2019). Alcohol use, a transdiagnostic risk factor for death by suicide, should be a routine part of any clinician's safety assessment. AUD elevates suicide risk by a factor of 10, and in the United States, a dose-response effect of alcohol intoxication raises the probability of firearm suicide in both men and women (Lange et al. 2023; Wilcox et al. 2004). AUD is a recognized potent factor of increased suicide risk independent of other disorders (Table 6–1).

The relationship between self-harm and suicide is complex. Self-harm is a reflection of deficits in symbolizing and expressing emotions through language (Gratz and Roemer 2008). The reliance on concrete strategies such as self-harm to release a sense of "badness" in the form of blood emerges more rapidly under the neurocognitive compromise of intoxication with alcohol (Gregory and Mustata 2012). NSSI has several functions, such as regulating negative emotions, decreasing numbness or emptiness, punishing the self, and communicating desperation (Nock and Prinstein 2004). Alcohol also increases impulsivity, aggravating self-harm (Links et al. 1995; Wilson et al. 2006). On a neurobiological level, self-injury is associated with abnormalities in brain regions associated with emotion, pain, reward, and interpersonal, self, and executive function processing (Brañas et al. 2021). NSSI may diminish inhibitions regarding suicidality via habituation of fear and pain, forming a so-called gateway to suicide (Hamza et al. 2012). Feeling disconnected from loved ones also increases suicide risk, which can be amplified by AUD pathology through various pathways (see next section and Table 2–2, Chapter 2).

This chapter focuses on clarifying the clinical management of NSSI and suicidal behavior in BPD+AUD. Using psychoeducation, infusing hope, and anchoring treatment in realistic goals, clinicians can change the patient's mind about their decision to engage in self-destructive behavior when urges arise. In good psychiatric management (GPM) broadly, clinicians aim to foster a sense of ownership by supporting independent decision-making and emphasizing a commitment to health and recovery even in challenging high-risk situations. GPM's interpersonal hypersensitivity (IHS) model serves as a framework to assess the current level of decompensation and provide strategies to address risk for self-harm versus suicide (see Figure 2–1 in Chapter 2). In the moment, risk assessment and judicious use of hospitalization are primary tools to ensure the pa-

Table 6–1. BPD and AUD: effects on suicidality and self-harm

Baseline	Suicide is the leading cause of death in people aged 15–34 years, and rates generally increase with age (Knipe et al. 2022).
	Self-injury is often a coping method, but it is strongly associated with suicidality (Favril et al. 2022).
	The prevalence of NSSI is 17.4% in adolescents, 13.4% in young adults, and 5.5% in adults (Swannell et al. 2014).
AUD	Alcohol use can cause disinhibition, aggressive behavior, and depressive symptoms (Hendler et al. 2011).
	Family conflict, interpersonal loss, unemployment, and legal problems are consequences of AUD (Perez et al. 2022).
	AUD is associated with a 94% increased risk of suicide (Isaacs et al. 2022).
	Alcohol contributes to enacting self-harm ideation (Melson and O'Connor, 2019). These instances typically encompass a spectrum ranging from unintentional overdoses to intentional self-harm, so it is crucial to investigate the presence of suicidality (Bohnert and Ilgen, 2019; Connery et al. 2022).
BPD	Suicide rates in BPD range from 3% to 10% (Paris and Zweig-Frank, 2001; Temes et al. 2019).
	Suicidal acts in BPD are usually ambivalent, and interpersonal connection decreases risk ("If rescued, I want to live. If not, I prefer to die").
	About 90% of individuals with BPD report self-harm (Goodman et al. 2017).
BPD + AUD	BPD + AUD patients can have higher lethality in suicide attempts (Wilson et al. 2006).
	Alcohol problems are often reported in the months prior to suicide in individuals with BPD (Flynn et al. 2020).

Note. AUD = alcohol use disorder; BPD = borderline personality disorder; NSSI = nonsuicidal self-injury.
Source. Adapted from Gunderson and Links 2014.

tient can survive the crisis; later, the clinician and patient can work collaboratively on how to reduce suicide risk. At the end of the chapter, common challenges in treatment are described, with concrete examples of how to apply GPM for BPD and AUD (GPM-AUD) principles to effectively work with BPD+AUD patients.

Formulation of Self-Harm and Suicide in the BPD+AUD Population

Deliberate self-harm occurs in the context of a stressful experience, often in interpersonal situations. Interpersonal sensitivity, low self-esteem, alcohol use, and social context transact in a way to promote instability in emotional processing and impulsivity for people with BPD. Emotional dysregulation and behavioral dyscontrol contribute to the development of BPD and AUD while also increasing risk for self-endangering behavior (Chesin et al. 2010; Chugani et al. 2020; Colmenero-Navarrete et al. 2022; Khemiri et al. 2016; MacKillop et al. 2022). GPM-AUD provides a cohesive framework for clinician and patient together to understand these factors, assess, and intervene effectively (see Figures 2–1 and 2–2).

Alcohol may serve many functions for patients, such as diminishing anxiety or stimulating positive affects (Hendler et al. 2011). As a means to cope over the long term, however, it worsens mood lability, impairs judgment, and leads to aggressive behavior (Mirijello et al. 2023). Adding AUD to BPD's broad instabilities can cause rapid deterioration toward dangerous behaviors. AUD also escalates stressful life problems (e.g., social isolation, conflicts, failure in attaining goals, loss of employment, and financial problems) that trigger both substance use and BPD symptoms. AUD increases acute risk of suicide (Borges et al. 2017) and reinforces the chronic and repeated cycles of interpersonal loss, damaged reputation, and self-esteem and the ongoing aloneness punctuated by intense moments of despair (Perez et al. 2022). Furthermore, alcohol misuse aggravates or perpetuates co-occurring disorders, such as depression (Yuodelis-Flores and Ries 2015), which in BPD is already prone to be more chronic and treatment resistant. Multiple relapses, ruptured attachments, and failures in self and interpersonal functioning accumulate in a vicious cycle to fuel two central motivators for suicide: thwarted belongingness and perceived burdensomeness (Van Orden et al. 2010).

Starting Treatment

Suicidal patients with BPD+AUD can be especially difficult to engage in treatment. They are stuck in ambivalence, skeptical that any treatment can be effective for them; some part of them wishes to die or feels they do not deserve to live. They may disown any interest in treatment, or they may display pathological dependence, wishing to be taken care of but passively resisting active engagement, focusing on how depressed and hopeless they feel, and continuing episodes of alcohol or drug intoxication. Treatment is more likely to be successful if the clinician can frame the first three or four sessions as "consultations" and spend time laying out a pathway to recovery, injecting hope, providing psychoeducation to align the patient with the tasks and goals of treatment, and fostering in the patient a sense of ownership for their own health and wellness.

Treatment Strategies to Target Underlying Vulnerabilities

Interpersonal Chain of Events and Emotional Processing

It can be difficult to reconstruct the events and emotions leading to a self-harm episode because of typical deficits in BPD related to identifying, acknowledging, and expressing emotions; associating them with related events; and reflecting on their practical and subjective consequences (Gregory and Remen 2008). During evaluation, inquire about feelings of rejection, shame, loneliness, self-criticism, and badness. Discuss who or what provided relief. Question the patient's understanding of their behaviors and the consequences of their actions. By being aware of behaviors and their impact on others and learning a more realistic understanding of relational dynamics, the patient can change dysfunctional relational patterns, regain agency, and shift from a hopeless sense of inherent badness to a sense of optimism and empowerment.

Patients might oppose these explorations out of shame, fear of rejection, or the need to maintain a sense of independent control. They may avoid discussion or omit important details about relapses or maladaptive behaviors. To effectively manage the patient's anxiety and build trust, when conducting the interview, a respectful and nonconfrontative approach is crucial.

Involving Patients in Safety Planning and Social Connection

A core principle of GPM is to enhance the patient's self-reliance as an antidote to their hypersensitivity to and dependence on others. GPM requires clinicians to involve patients in managing their own safety by asking the patient's opinion on possible solutions or what they could have done in the past in a similar situation, rather than trying to control the patient or give praise when they "did the right thing" (Gregory and Mustata 2012). Although BPD patients might protest and be frustrated, this process normalizes the disappointing reality that one's personal safety cannot depend on the availability of others, and instead empowers them to have a plan of action to cope through despairing or desperate moments while asking others for the support they need. Clinicians can validate the wish to have someone care for them when they feel suicidal, while avoiding the need for unsustainable heroic measures that only reinforce idealization and passive hopes for rescue.

Safety plans are a standard of care in self-harm management (Stanley and Brown 2012). The construction of the plan involves "rewinding" maladaptive behaviors and events to identify triggers, warning signs, coping skills, and helpful interpersonal contacts and thereby create a safer environment (Table 6–2). By engaging in this process, patients learn about their functioning and how to handle future stressors (see section "Think First" in Chapter 2). After self-harm episodes occur, it is important to review the safety plan even if patients complain about it being repetitive. If the patient persists in self-harm and reckless behavior, agreement on the safety plan as a central requirement of the treatment goals will be crucial to maintaining the clinical framework of care (see later section, "Treatment Challenges").

Clinicians can involve the patient in generating alternative ways of coping with situations that trigger drinking (relapse prevention) or deliberate self-harm. Engage in problem-solving ("Thinking about this now, was there anything you could have done differently?") and reflect on what the patient learned from the experience. Some patients may initially rely on you to resolve crises, but it is essential to foster their autonomy while still validating their struggles. Likewise, in the treatment of substance use disorders, a critical component of relapse prevention is to build self-efficacy through learning from relapse episodes and creating new strategies to cope using healthier behaviors.

It is important to remember that patients generally are ambivalent about treatment, and this manifests in symptom recurrence, missed appointments, and relapses. Improvement of symptoms can be threatening, because patients fear losing support if their symptoms resolve. Be skeptical of passive compliance (the patient mechanically follows every treatment task from the beginning or does not give any input), because this indicates that the patient is not fully engaging in treatment planning. To buffer rejection sensitivity, say that you appreciate how hard it is to

Table 6–2. Example safety plan

Step	Examples
Step 1: Warning signs	Anxious and restless Want to go to a bar or drink alone Angry
Step 2: Coping strategies	Listen to music or podcast Play basketball or go for a walk Play a video game or do a puzzle Log in to a virtual mutual-help meeting
Step 3: Social ways to distract or connect	Go to the café next door Call friends [include names and numbers] Go to a live mutual-help meeting
Step 4: Ways to ask for help	Talk to spouse Text AA sponsor [include number] Call recovery buddy [include number]
Step 5: Professional help or agencies	Clinician's office [include number] Suicide prevention line (988) Local emergency department [include number]
Step 6: Ways to make environment safe	Do not keep pills in stock at home Do not keep alcohol or other drugs at home Remove all firearms from home

Source.   Adapted from Stanley and Brown 2012.

change, and you hope to continue working together toward recovery in the face of setbacks. Occasionally reframe expectations to bolster alliance by emphasizing the patient's role in effective treatment. This empowers the patient to choose the path to recovery.

Involving Family and Friends

Clinicians will often need to talk with patients' loved ones in times of suicidal crisis, and this should be discussed at the start of treatment when expectations, roles, and goals are established. Highlight how insight and judgment may be altered in the moment, and so treatment depends on planning ahead. When the patient struggles to think clearly, the family can provide nonreactive support or help the patient connect with professional help. Families need support and psychoeducation about the clinician's abilities and limitations; the family may need additional support to prevent burnout and depression (see section "Support for Family Members" in Chapter 8; see also Appendix C).

Families can play a key role in making the home environment less stressful and more safe, and thus reduce risk of patient self-harm. Educate families about how to protect against alcohol relapse and suicide. Provide psychoeducation about the IHS model of GPM, when leaning in versus unilateral action is optimal, and how to avoid being motivated solely by the patient's anger. Involving the family prevents the clinician from being idealized as a source of rescue, and also relieves the clinician from bearing unrealistic responsibility for the patient's safety.

Suicide Risk Assessment

First, evaluate immediate threats to safety. Superficial NSSI or transient suicidal thoughts in the context of feeling threatened are not as dangerous as impulsive self-damaging behaviors that patients resort to when they are disconnected from others, dissociated, intoxicated, or in despair. Inflating the concern over nondangerous behaviors may needlessly escalate the level of care and decrease the patient's agency (i.e., a sense of ownership of their own treatment and recovery).

GPM-AUD relies on usual methods of assessing suicide risk in line with the general mental health training most clinicians receive (Gold et al. 2020). Suicide attempts associated with BPD and AUD are often ambivalent (e.g., "If rescued, I want to live; if not, then I want to die"). Patients have layers of acuity that emerge in stressful situations on top of preexisting chronic risk factors of suicide. Therefore, the traditional acute-on-chronic risk model (Links et al. 2003) is helpful to assess chronically suicidal patients, indicating risk changes typical for these patients (Figure 6–1).

It is essential to monitor current increases in alcohol and substance use, persistent intoxication, recent adverse life events, changes in psychosocial status, relapse, withdrawal symptoms, severe agitation, anxiety, insomnia, burdensomeness, and depression (Lamis and Malone, 2011; Modesto-Lowe et al. 2006; Perez et al. 2022). The availability of means for suicide (e.g., firearms, medication) should always be evaluated (Ryan and Oquendo 2020). Other ways to reduce risk are supporting sobriety, including 12-step and other recovery support groups (Esang and Ahmed 2018), and managing intense emotional interactions while helping patients describe and integrate their experiences (Gregory and Remen 2008).

Acute exacerbation of risk

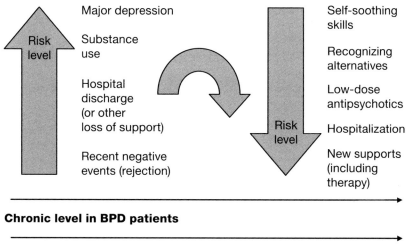

Figure 6–1.   Acute-on-chronic suicide risk.

Note.   BPD = borderline personality disorder.
Source.   Gunderson and Links 2014. Used with permission.

Involving Other Colleagues, Limitations, and Liability

Clinicians may be stressed and feel helpless when dealing with suicide risk (Menon et al. 2020). Negative countertransference reactions might be substantial (Gabbard 1993). Supervision, consultation, and team meetings to discuss difficult cases to gain support all help clinicians to think more clearly about effective interventions with the support of colleagues who can relate to the stressful dilemmas of working with high-risk, complex patients. Evidence-based specialist therapies for BPD include in their structure regular consultation groups to provide space, support, and structure for processing the many emotional and interpersonal challenges of working with patients who are self-destructive, as a measure to increase clinical effectiveness and reduce clinician burnout.

Clearly, clinicians want to save patients from catastrophic outcomes such as suicide, but our current ability to predict self-harm has serious limitations (Knipe et al. 2022). We cannot forecast with high certainty

whether patients will recall and implement their safety plans or whether
they'll face other dangerous situations in their everyday lives. Clinicians
therefore may feel helpless, uncertain, and powerless, which can increase
anxiety, stressful arousal, and action without reflection. Being broadly
available might reduce these uncertain and helpless feelings, but in reality, clinicians cannot be 100% available. Working with realistic limitations
and honestly communicating them is appropriate when establishing the
treatment framework, so that the conversation does not originate in the
moment of crisis. If the clinician were to propose excessive availability,
they would be reinforcing idealization and dependence, working against
the major goals of patient responsibility and autonomy in BPD treatment.

In some countries, clinicians must worry about litigation and liability
(Gunderson and Links 2014). Guidelines exist to navigate these situations, and clinicians should know the standards of care that relate to their
professional discipline, locally and nationally. Obtaining second opinions and perspectives from colleagues can also ensure that treatment is
appropriate and has low risk of litigation (Table 6–3).

Levels of Care

The outpatient setting is the most effective context for the treatment of
BPD+AUD unless the patient needs withdrawal management from alcohol or has co-occurring disorders that require residential level of care to
achieve stabilization (see Chapter 9, "Level-of-Care Considerations").
The proper level of care should be chosen to further the goal of the patient being able to deal with their relationships, triggers, and emotions in
their everyday lives.

The availability of higher levels of care, such as day treatment (partial
hospital services) or residential treatment, can lessen the use of emergency and inpatient services, as well as serve as a stabilizing transition
back to successful outpatient care (Figure 6–2). Unfortunately, these options are not widely available, leaving many patients in a cycle between
outpatient appointments, emergency room evaluations, and inpatient
hospitalizations. Outpatient strategies to avoid unnecessary disruptions
in care include expanding the patient's social network (see Chapter 8,
"Multimodal Treatments") with use of family supports, mutual help
groups, and other nontreatment activities that broker positive relationships with others in sober contexts.

When considering hospitalization, clinicians should always balance
benefits (e.g., safety) and risks (e.g., iatrogenic life avoidance) (Vijay and

Table 6–3. Liability concerns regarding self-endangering behaviors in patients with BPD

The risk of liability is low (<1%) and lessens with therapist experience.

Poor management of the clinician-patient relationship increases the risk of liability. Pay attention to countertransference enactments such as unrealistic availability, punitive hostility, personal involvement, and illusions of omniscience or omnipotence.

To minimize liability:

• Ensure careful documentation, mainly risk assessments and clinical decisions (Packman et al. 2004; Paris 2004).

• Discuss and consult with colleagues or split treatments (Gunderson and Links 2014).

• Involve the patient's family in psychoeducation (e.g., how suicidality occurs, suicide rates) and suicidal management (e.g., warning signs) (Gutheil 2004).

• Establish a healthy relationship with the patient's family (Packman et al. 2004).

• Show support for the patient's family after suicidal behavior (Gutheil 2004).

Note. BPD = borderline personality disorder.
Source. Adapted from Gunderson and Links 2014.

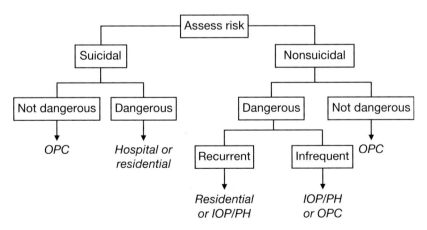

Figure 6–2. Algorithm to select the level of care in response to self-endangering behaviors.

Note. IOP = intensive outpatient; OPC = outpatient clinic/office practice; PH = partial hospital.
Source. Gunderson and Links 2014. Used with permission.

Links 2007). Short stays (1–14 days) are desirable, as longer stays allow patients to passively avoid life challenges. To make inpatient stays more effective, focus on understanding the stressors the patient was not able to cope with and collaboratively develop strategies to address them after discharge. This requires active outpatient clinician collaboration with the teams at this higher level of care. Inpatient stays are also an opportunity to reevaluate psychopharmacology agents and increase family support. The risk of suicide increases immediately after discharge, so a gradual transition from inpatient to partial hospital, residential, and intensive outpatient treatment can decrease stress of the process for patients and help troubleshoot difficulties. Communicate with the inpatient or acute care staff to coordinate the discharge plan.

Treatment Challenges

Death From Suicide

Suicides are devastating for families and friends. Everyone wonders what could have been done to prevent it.

When death by suicide occurs, the first step is to consider informing authorities, clinical staff, and family members. The last interaction with the patient should be carefully documented. Also, suggest meeting with the family to listen and assist them in understanding what happened. Most families appreciate this effort. Family members who have suffered a loss by suicide are themselves at increased risk for mental health disorders (e.g., PTSD or depression), and support can be provided for connection to treatment if indicated.

A patient's death by suicide is devastating for clinicians as well (Goldblatt et al. 2020); it is an inherent risk in our profession and cannot always be prevented. After such a loss, the clinician should debrief and process the loss with colleagues (Sakinofsky 2007). Psychological autopsies or formal postmortem meetings can expand perspectives and support learning—as long as the emphasis is on mutual support and learning, rather than finger-pointing.

Evidence suggests that "postvention" discussions help manage the catastrophic loss of suicide (Andriessen et al. 2019a). Although no established guidelines exist, social support and education can be beneficial (Andriessen et al. 2019b). The American Foundation for Suicide Prevention website has tools and a support group search engine (https://afsp.org).

Frequent Crisis Phone Calls

Guidelines should be made at the start of therapy for between-session contact (see section "Intersession Availability" in Chapter 5). Communication between sessions should be for urgent matters only and should be rare—for example, consider limiting the frequency of contacts to twice a week or less. Otherwise, there is a risk of clinician burnout. To prevent feelings of rejection down the road, explain this limit to the patient at the start of therapy:

> Given everything that is going on, I understand that meeting weekly may not be enough, and you may need support at times I cannot be available. Can we consider adding other group activities to your schedule?

Any between-session contact should be documented, discussed, and explored during the next session. Work with patients to create a support network so that they attempt other steps in their safety plan before calling on clinical professionals for assistance. Remind patients that a part of treatment is learning to rely more on themselves and less on therapists or other caregivers. If excessive calls or messaging continue, revisit the guidelines set out at the start of treatment. Focus on identifying emotions related to the calls and not being able to access the clinician as often as desired. Create a plan with the patient for when they may call the therapist and when they should rely on other supports.

The Patient Does Not Want to Go to the Emergency Department or Hospital When Advised

If the patient poses a significant threat to self or others, assess risk mindfully. Review the initial agreement from the start of treatment about the patient's commitment to keeping themselves safe; remind them that you can be helpful only if they work toward safety and recovery. Gently and empathetically point out that your ability to be beneficial at the moment is impaired, knowing that the patient is not safe enough. Emphasize that after the crisis is resolved, you would like them to come back to resume treatment.

> If I do nothing right now, you will feel uncared for by me. But if I send you to the ER against your will, you will feel disrespected by me. Either way, your refusal to keep yourself safe jeopardizes our relationship and your treatment.

This intervention puts the dilemma back on the patient and helps to preserve the therapeutic alliance, regardless of whether you decide to hospitalize the patient involuntarily.

Self-Harm During a Regular Appointment

Any self-harm in a session must be dealt with supportively and directly. Say, "Self-harm during sessions is not permitted. The sessions are about learning to put your experiences into words instead of self-harming." Remind the patient that not resorting to these behaviors is a goal of treatment.

Use of self-harm when the clinician is available signals a problem in the treatment relationship. Once the behaviors have stopped, explore the associated emotions and thoughts before the incident occurred. If the behaviors continue despite intervention, the session should end early. Ensure that the patient has a safe disposition.

The Patient Refuses to Be Discharged

The hospital setting can be a soothing but regressive environment for patients with BPD. As a rule, patients can be discharged by demonstrating a lessening in self-harm thinking and better judgment; however, in patients with BPD, these criteria may send the message that if they improve, they will no longer be cared for. Because of this intense fear, patients with BPD will often negatively react to the "threat" of discharge, possibly increasing suicidal ideation. Explain that these behaviors are signs that hospitalization may harm them, and therefore it would be in their best interest to resume outpatient treatment instead. A discharge date (or a specific goal) can be set at the start of hospitalization to limit expectations about the length of stay. Warn patients about the dangers of hospitalization and the potential for symptoms to deteriorate; discharge should be sooner than later if decompensation occurs. Responsible, minimal reliance on hospitalization is a treatment goal.

The Patient Does Not Disclose a Suicide Attempt

Review treatment expectations and inquire about the patient's commitment to pursue health and recovery, including keeping themselves safe. Next, explore the reasons for not disclosing the suicide attempt, which may be associated with intense shame, anger, or humiliation. It is important to examine stressors in the clinician-patient relationship (e.g., vacation). The clinician might feel a sense of helplessness or that they care more about the patient's health than the patient does; be careful not to trigger shame about the attempt. If shame is discussed, it can be helpful to point out that this is a complex feeling that also signals how the patient does care about their behavior and choices.

Chronic Suicidality and Alcohol Intoxication

Chronic suicidality should be differentiated from acute suicidal ideation (Paris 2002). There are two concerns in these cases: chronic suicidality and a potential trigger for acute suicidality: namely, alcohol. Instead of telling a patient to stop a specific behavior such as drinking, explore the positive and negative aspects of the behavior (function and consequences), including the impact of drinking on suicidal ideation. Use this opportunity to discuss working toward health, recovery, and a treatment plan beyond suicidal thoughts. Remember to be nonjudgmental.

From a risk evaluation perspective, overestimating danger may lead to iatrogenic consequences (e.g., hospitalizing a patient who is asking for help). To be dismissive or frustrated with a patient can escalate risk; patients already feel ashamed of their actions.

It can be difficult to explore the reasons for continuous drinking in these situations. The patient may deny that alcohol is a problem, externalize the problem, or blame interpersonal issues to avoid inner conflict and shame. For example, they may say, "My drinking is not a problem. It's my boss who won't get off my back about it and always threatens to fire me! He's the problem, not me!" Make statements that help internalize the conflict, such as, "Do you sometimes feel you and the drinking are the problems at your work? Are there times you feel this way?" Provide psychoeducation on the functions of suicidality and the risks of continued drinking in such circumstances.

For collaborative patients, help create a personalized scale to rate their safety and appropriate contacts if safety concerns worsen (acute suicidality). This process promotes agency, lessens all-or-none thinking, and helps identify acute ideation.

Persistent Nonsuicidal Self-Injury

NSSI relieves the tension of unprocessed emotions and helps to limit interpersonal stress by turning the anger onto the self, preserving relationships for a bit longer. If the patient continues to persist in NSSI, remind them of their commitment to health and recovery. Help them assess the risks and benefits of self-harm and its consequences. Address shame sources, offer understanding for abandonment or rejection fears, and promote acceptance of anger.

NSSI can resurface, signaling ambivalence about recovery. Be wary of clinician and patient fantasies of being able to control the self-injurious behaviors, as this may be the patient attempting to avoid internal conflict by bringing conflict and control struggles into the therapeutic relationship. As patients improve their ability to manage their inner conflicts and start to see others in a more integrated way (less black-and-white thinking), they also feel less certainty about their interactions with others, triggering distress.

Relapse into self-injury may also be related to grief about getting well and being less reliant on others in a sick role. Improvement can seem intimidating: if they improve, they may lose support or be abandoned by caregivers. If self-harm fails to respond to interventions, focus on life-building goals.

Suicidal When Intoxicated But Does Not Remember

Patients frequently present to the emergency department because of suicidal ideation or threat related to intoxication. This is distressing for loved ones. Provide psychoeducation about alcohol's effects on mood, anxiety, and self-harm thinking. Help patients weigh the pros and cons of their behavior, for example, "I know you mentioned that drinking helps quite a bit with anxiety, but I wonder if your family being worried about you ending up in the emergency room because of suicidal thoughts causes even more anxiety." If the patient denies the problem, say, "I know that now you are feeling fine, but last Saturday you sent me an email saying that life was not worth it. Don't you think this is something important?"

Drinking to Death and Indifference Toward Safety

Some patients may indirectly put themselves and others in dangerous situations by their alcohol intoxication, binge drinking, and engaging in risky behaviors such as drinking and driving. Although there is no explicit suicidal ideation, the recklessness of their behavior prompts questions about suicidal fantasies or indifference toward death (Miller 2009). Additionally, some patients use other substances (e.g., opioids) compulsively and may overdose. Evaluating suicidality in these circumstances is essential (Connery et al. 2022). Recount an interpersonal chain of events, involving them in their safety and assessing risk, for example, "You are saying that you are okay, but let's review what happened last week when you had that accident." Offer nonreactive support that does not praise sobriety or shame drinking or relapses. Normalize that while you can be of support, sobriety and safety depend on the patient.

The Patient Is Not Fully Participating in Treatment or Is in a Passive Suicide Ideation State

Reassure the patient that you're there to collaborate with them, and they need to remain actively engaged instead of sitting back passively waiting to be cured. This instills hope and a sense that the condition is treatable, encouraging the patient to work through and resolve issues rather than seeking a quick fix from the therapist. Example:

> *Patient:* You cannot make me want to live. I will not go to the ER, because life is meaningless.
>
> *Therapist:* I understand that a part of you wants to die, but we can only be helpful if you decide you want to recover. I realize recovery is difficult. I understand that if you choose otherwise, there's nothing we can do to stop you. But if you decide you want to work toward recovery, I think you are capable of doing that, you are capable of getting into a better place, and I would love to work with you in that direction.

Conclusion

Self-harm and suicidality are diagnostic of BPD when occurring in the context of interpersonal and emotional instability. Self-destructive tendencies are of particular concern when they co-occur with AUD, which increases disinhibition and neurocognitive compromise. Putting these behaviors in their interpersonal context helps patients more effectively process their emotions and feelings. An assessment of danger and acute risk guides the selection of appropriate level of care and interventions. Ultimately, as with GPM's approach more broadly, safety management aims to reinforce the patient's sense of responsibility over their own behavior and treatment while providing the support to do so more effectively and constructively over time.

7

Pharmacotherapy for Co-occurring Borderline Personality Disorder and Alcohol Use Disorder

Carl Fleisher, M.D.
Jeffrey DeVido, M.D.

Diagnostic complexity is the rule rather than the exception for individuals with bordeline personality disorder (BPD). Studies demonstrate the high co-occurrence of BPD and alcohol use disorder (AUD), with approximately half of those diagnosed with BPD also meeting criteria for AUD, and 14%–17% of those with current AUD also meeting criteria for BPD (Trull et al. 2000; 20182018).

Clinically, this degree of co-occurrence is of little surprise. The effects of alcohol misuse impair mental health broadly. Early-onset alcohol use disorder bears developmental consequences, as symptoms interfere with stable formation of personality functioning during critical periods of adolescence and young adulthood (Spear 2018). Socially relevant emotions such as shame, anger, and anxiety are triggers for alcohol use; these same emotions arise from the interpersonal hypersensitivity in people with BPD. Intense emotions can emerge for social reasons, such as conflict in significant relationships, poor self-esteem, or setting aside personal desires to please others—a dynamic that typically breeds anger, unhappiness, and resentment.

Although social and emotional factors drive both BPD and AUD, medical interventions that are standard of care for AUD are frequently underutilized. This chapter reviews current evidence-based practice for the medical management of AUD and contextualizes implementation for patients with co-occurring BPD.

Principles

We offer eight principles to keep in mind when treating this common clinical profile (Table 7–1).

First, it is critical to address these disorders simultaneously. Sequential approaches ("treat this, then that") or parallel treatments ("I treat this, you treat that," aka "split treatment") are common yet inferior to integrated care (the care team delivers evidence-based therapeutic interventions for both disorders) with respect to improvement of mental health symptoms (Chetty et al. 2023). Thus, integrated care is always preferred.

If integrated care is unavailable, parallel care services may be more effective when clinicians collaborate closely to deliver care and assess outcomes. Clinicians skilled in treating AUD may lack training in treating BPD, and vice versa (Gregory et al. 2022), and availability of services to treat BPD or AUD is often inadequate. Of note, the original version of good psychiatric management (GPM) for BPD (Gunderson and Links 2014) strongly encouraged sobriety before addressing alcohol or other substance use disorders (SUDs); this manual aims to update the GPM model to be consistent with current evidence-based strategies for simultaneous treatment of BPD+AUD without contingencies for achieving sobriety first.

The second principle of treating BPD+AUD is to **establish the framework** of treatment. GPM, as a pragmatic approach, borrows from the two common frameworks of treating AUD, namely the medical model and the 12-step recovery model. GPM for BPD and AUD (GPM-AUD) borrows two concepts from the medical model. First, patients are described as having illnesses that they do not control but that they are responsible for addressing. This is a foundation for promoting agency. Second, medications ought to be prescribed based on current care standards for each disorder. GPM-AUD also borrows two tangible components of the 12-step recovery model. First, patients join with each other in *fellowship*. Joining others combats the isolation frequently felt by those with AUD and BPD. Patients with BPD have likewise been shown to ben-

Table 7–1. Principles of co-occurring treatment

1. Address BPD and AUD simultaneously.
2. Set framework, including parts of medical and 12-step models.
3. Safety is top priority.
4. Keep patients in treatment.
5. Encourage autonomy.
6. Prescribe medication based on standards of care, not countertransference.
7. Negotiate for behavior change.
8. Avoid polypharmacy.

Note. AUD=alcohol use disorder; BPD=borderline personality disorder.

efit from participating in various kinds of groups. Second, patients are expected to take a moral, emotional *inventory*. We encourage this task as one that is both active and self-reflective.

The third principle is that **safety is the top priority**. Alcohol use can threaten patients' health acutely and severely, so clinicians ought to proactively encourage medications indicated for alcohol reduction or cessation. This stands in contrast to pharmacotherapy for BPD, which lacks an evidence base (Leichsenring et al. 2023). A general approach to BPD pharmacotherapy is to provide standard treatment for all co-occurring disorders (such as depressive and anxiety disorders, ADHD, PTSD, and other SUDs), plus limited use of medications to address the symptoms, behaviors, or states that cause the greatest impairment in functioning or safety (such as insomnia or emotional crisis).

Fourth, it is **vital to keep patients in treatment**. To maximize the likelihood of successful treatment, clinicians must nurture the therapeutic relationship and prescribe medications that are effective for symptom relief, thereby improving treatment retention. Of note, GPM originally recommended that treaters terminate care in the absence of functional progress. With co-occurring AUD, however, we make a distinction: how long the patient remains in active treatment is a meaningful measure of progress and is itself a good outcome.

The fifth principle is to **encourage patient autonomy**. Make clear that treatment is always voluntary and collaborative. When encouraging a medication trial, educate and explain the potential risks and benefits, respectfully accept the patient's decision to try medication or not, and clearly document the informed consent discussion. Treaters must navigate the fine line between using medications to treat a medical illness

(AUD) and emphasizing self-care, while not falling into the trap of rein-forcing an overly medicalized view in which patients see AUD as something that controls them (where the individual has no power and therefore no agency to address the illness). When a patient agrees to a medication trial, educate them about what target symptoms they should be tracking and emphasize that medication adherence is critical. Clinicians are most helpful when they use a clear, predictable, and structured assessment of how and when a patient is taking or missing prescribed doses, whether the trial is tolerable, and which target symptoms are improving.

Consistent with this frame, we encourage treaters to adopt *neuroscience-based nomenclature*. For instance, valproic acid, formerly called a mood stabilizer, is termed a histone deacetylase inhibitor. This nomenclature may help prevent patients and treaters alike from falling into the trap of label-based prescribing (e.g., mood stabilizers for unstable mood, antidepressants for sadness and suicidality). A glossary of neuroscience based terms is available for download at https://nbn2r.com/authors. As another strategy to encourage autonomy, treaters can promote self-efficacy in parallel with any pharmacotherapy—that is, treaters can nurture a mindset of "I am taking action to treat my medical illness" (referring to AUD).

Sixth, treaters must **prescribe medication based on standards of care, not countertransference**. By this we mean to discourage prescribing medication to satisfy anyone's emotional needs—the clinician's or the patient's. Patients' needs typically involve requesting medications as a way to lessen distress. Treaters' needs may vary: to garner appreciation, to dispel fear, to feel pride in helping the patient, to reduce stress or confusion (if not sure what else to do), to save time (if prescribing seems more expedient than therapy), or to avoid insisting that patients tolerate distress, and hence avoiding potential disagreement or disappointment from the patient.

If a medication offers genuine value, the treater can prescribe it and then assess the value within a set time. The value of each medication should be reassessed at least quarterly. Value can be measured in the short or long term. Regardless, the duration of the medication trial should correspond to the duration of its value.

If patients request medication, treaters need not reflexively discourage it, but instead should aim to be thoughtful about the anticipated value of that intervention. Discuss the pros and cons of medication. Explain your point of view and inquire respectfully about the patient's point of view. Conversely, if treaters recommend medication and patients initially decline, again the aim is to be thoughtful. The essential point is not whether the medication gets prescribed, but how treaters and patients arrive at their decision.

Seventh, treaters should **negotiate for behavioral change** whenever possible. If the patient starts a medication trial, suggest that it be paired with actions that support abstinence (or reduced drinking) and promote self-care. Patients could be asked to learn about their illness, attend a 12-step or other mutual-help program, make measurable progress toward one of the 12 steps, or practice a BPD coping skill. Teach that the role of medications is to support the behavioral treatment program.

The eighth and final principle is to **avoid polypharmacy and limit "as needed" or "prn" prescribing**. The various medications for AUD rely on different mechanisms of action, so it may be tempting to consider combining them in the hopes of deriving additional benefit. The current literature does not support such an approach, however, with very limited exceptions (e.g., initiating maintenance AUD treatments concurrently with shorter-term withdrawal management medications; disulfiram plus acamprosate in one small study) (Anton et al. 2006). Similarly, among patients with BPD, polypharmacy is inversely associated with outcome (i.e., more medications track with worse outcomes) (Shapiro-Thompson and Fineberg 2022). Research has not shown that any medication or class of medications consistently benefits patients with BPD (Table 7–2). No national regulatory body (FDA or European Medicines Agency) has approved any medication to treat the symptoms of BPD. It is important to avoid prn medication schedules because both BPD and AUD patients are vulnerable to impulsive self-dosing or dose escalation when experiencing distress (Figure 7–1). If there is a transient need for medication adjunct, prescribe it on a fixed dose interval and educate the patient on the dangers of dose escalation or schedule changes, particularly if they continue to consume alcohol. Select medications that are safely compatible with alcohol use and avoid medications with significant negative or dangerous interaction. In most cases, benzodiazepine use is discouraged, because it interferes with learning and may lead to aggressive self-harm or violent behaviors when combined with alcohol (Linnoila 1990).

Pharmacotherapy

Repeated use of alcohol (or other substances) causes various adaptations—neurobiological, psychological, and physiological—that favor continued use. This section is organized around first, those adaptations

Table 7–2.   Current status of pharmacotherapy for BPD

Approximately 35 randomized controlled trials have been conducted (dopamine receptor antagonists, serotonin and/or norepinephrine reuptake inhibitors, glutamatergic agents, and others), usually with small samples (average $N = 40$), variable outcome measures, and limited duration.

No medication is uniformly or dramatically helpful.

No drug has been licensed by the FDA as an effective treatment for BPD.

Research sponsored by pharmaceutical companies has been limited by disproportionate fears of violent or suicidal acts in patients who receive or do not receive medications (and the resulting liability).

Polypharmacy is associated with multiple side effects, and the effects of augmentation are unknown.

The number of medications taken is inversely related to improvement.

Minimal attention has been given to the effects of medication on interpersonal relationships.

Note.   BPD = borderline personality disorder; FDA = Food and Drug Administration.
Source.   Adapted from Gunderson and Links 2014.

that require acute pharmacotherapeutic management (i.e., withdrawal management pharmacotherapies), and second, those adaptations that result in the behavior changes leading to chronic continued use of alcohol that are the hallmark of AUD (i.e., maintenance AUD pharmacotherapies). These two adaptations have significant overlap, but it is nonetheless useful to consider them distinctly, because there are different clinical risks and considerations in each of these phases (Table 7–3).

Withdrawal Management

Chronic alcohol use can result in neurobiological and physiological adaptations manifesting as the phenomena of tolerance (a person needs to consume a greater quantity of alcohol to achieve the same effect) and withdrawal (hyperarousal symptoms such as tremor, sweating, nausea, increased heart rate and blood pressure, and anxiety). The body's response to alcohol can be seen as a constant struggle to maintain balance between the inhibitory effects of alcohol and the body's own excitatory systems—the body will adapt to the presence of chronic alcohol exposure by upregulating its excitatory systems (i.e., glutamatergic and sympathetic pathways) and downregulating its inhibitory systems (i.e., GABAergic pathways). Tolerance is the result of adaptations in the glutamatergic, sympathetic, and GABAergic pathways. Alcohol withdrawal

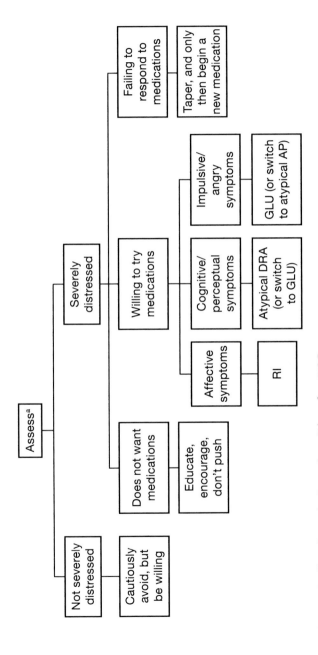

Figure 7–1. Medication choice algorithm for BPD.

Note. BPD=borderline personality disorder; DRA=dopamine receptor antagonist; GLU=glutamatergic agent such as valproic acid or lamotrigine; RI=reuptake inhibitor (serotonin and/or norepinephrine).

[a]Assess 1) patient motivation; 2) symptom severity and type: anxiety/depression/affective instability, impulsive/anger, cognitive/perceptual; and 3) current medications. If patient is severely distressed or insistent, proceed as follows: 1) affectively unstable, anxious/depressed: start with GLU (e.g., topiramate or lamotrigine), move to RI; 2) impulsive/anger: start with DRA (e.g., aripiprazole or ziprasidone) or GLU, move to the other class of medication; 3) cognitive/perceptual: start with DRA, move to other types.

Source. Adapted from Gunderson and Links 2014.

Table 7-3.　Symptom targets and medication types

	Mood instability	Depression	Anxiety	Anger	Impulsivity	Cognitive/ perceptual
Selective serotonin reuptake inhibitors	?	+	?	?	+	–
Tricyclic antidepressants	–	–	–	+	?	–
Glutamatergic agents	+	?/+	?	++	++	–
Dopamine receptor antagonists	+	?	+	+	+	++
Anxiolytics	?	–	?	–	–	?

Note.　++ = helpful; + = modestly helpful; ? = uncertain; – = negative.
Source.　Gunderson and Links 2014; adapted from Mercer et al. 2009; Silk and Faurino 2012.

manifests when alcohol consumption abruptly ceases or is significantly curtailed. Withdrawal is characterized by overexcitation due to upregulated glutamatergic and sympathetic pathways that have not yet had a chance to rebalance in the absence of alcohol. Many factors (e.g., genetics, gender, duration and volume of alcohol use, certain medical conditions) can contribute to the speed and severity of tolerance development.

Alcohol withdrawal can present on a spectrum of severity from mild (tremors, anxiety, and insomnia) to severe (seizures or autonomic instability—i.e., hyperthermia, delirium, hypertensive crisis, aka delirium tremens). Severe alcohol withdrawal may be life threatening and warrants emergency care. Withdrawal requires medical assessment and often (depending on severity) pharmacotherapy and hospitalization. The physiology of alcohol tolerance and withdrawal is independent of whether one has BPD or other mental health disorders.

Pharmacotherapies for alcohol withdrawal management are best understood using the model of excitatory/inhibitory imbalance described earlier. Pharmacotherapies aim to restore balance in a safe, controlled manner, specifically through two methods. First, benzodiazepine receptor agonists and allosteric modulators of the GABA-A receptor (e.g., phenobarbital) enhance the endogenous inhibitory pathways that have been downregulated through chronic alcohol exposure; they may be thought of as medications that fully substitute for alcohol but are dosed to minimize intoxication effects. These medication classes comprise the most widely used approach to withdrawal management of AUD. Second, glutamatergic agents, including voltage-gated sodium and calcium channel blockers (e.g., valproate, carbamazepine, or gabapentin) quiet the excitatory pathways that were upregulated by chronic alcohol exposure and provide alternate options to benzodiazepine and barbiturate taper schedules.

Alcohol withdrawal pharmacotherapies can be administered in either outpatient or inpatient settings, depending on clinical assessment of risk of severe withdrawal. To determine the appropriateness of inpatient versus outpatient treatment, first screen for alcohol use (e.g., Alcohol Use Disorders Identification Test-Piccinelli Consumption [AUDIT-PC]; see Appendix E), conduct a physical examination, and obtain a comprehensive clinical history. If obtaining a history is difficult owing to patient intoxication, seek collateral information from close supports. It is useful to obtain a basic comprehensive metabolic panel and hepatic panel; however, urgent treatment may be required before results can be assessed. If a patient in the outpatient setting is not acutely intoxicated, it is helpful to ask if they have had any nondrinking days within the past 30 days, and if yes, whether any symptoms of alcohol withdrawal were present.

The American Society of Addiction Medicine (ASAM) published useful clinical guidelines for alcohol withdrawal assessment and treatment in 2020. The guidelines, summarized in Table 7–4, highlight the risk factors for a patient to develop severe alcohol withdrawal that may warrant inpatient treatment.

Inpatient pharmacotherapy approaches to treating alcohol withdrawal generally fall into two categories. The first is symptom-triggered, in which medications are administered in response to emerging symptoms of withdrawal. Withdrawal is assessed through a validated screening tool such as the Clinical Institute Withdrawal Assessment-Alcohol, Revised (CIWA-Ar; Sullivan et al. 1989) (see Appendix E). Benzodiazepines are typically prescribed, for example, lorazepam 1–2 mg every 1–2 hours as needed. (Note that as-needed prescribing is acceptable in the inpatient setting, since treaters can supervise medication use.) The second approach is a front-loaded, fixed-dose approach. In this approach, prescribers typically give benzodiazepines such as chlordiazepoxide 50–100 mg every 1–2 hours for three doses. Once the patient's symptoms are stable, medication is then tapered over several days. Among inpatients with severe alcohol withdrawal, benzodiazepine receptor agonists and allosteric modulators of the GABA-A receptor are typically loaded as a 10 mg/kg intravenous dose, infused over 30 minutes, or a 60–260 mg oral or intramuscular dose. Often, treaters coadminister glutamatergic agents (e.g., gabapentin 1,200 mg loading dose; carbamazepine 600–800 mg total per day) or adrenergic blocking medications (e.g., clonidine).

Outpatient management may be appropriate when the clinician judges the patient to be at low risk of severe alcohol withdrawal. The key to successful outpatient treatment is close contact between the patient and the treater or clinic. Close contact ensures that treaters can manage symptoms dynamically, based on emerging needs. In particular, clinicians should monitor for symptom escalation, because escalation despite optimal outpatient pharmacotherapy can indicate that a higher level of care is warranted. Withdrawal severity should be assessed over time using validated tools. This can be done either in-person with the CIWA-Ar or, in more reliable patients, with self-report scales such as the Short Alcohol Withdrawal Scale (SAWS; Gossop et al. 2002) (see Appendix E). Sample outpatient alcohol withdrawal regimens are shown in Figure 7–2.

Table 7–4. Clinical guidelines for alcohol withdrawal assessment and treatment in an inpatient, medically monitored setting

History of delirium or seizure with alcohol withdrawal

Numerous withdrawal episodes in the patient's lifetime

Comorbid medical or surgical illness (especially traumatic brain injury)

Older age (>65 years)

Long duration of heavy and regular alcohol consumption

Seizure during the current withdrawal episode

Marked autonomic hyperactivity on presentation

Physiological dependence on GABAergic agents such as benzodiazepines or barbiturates

Source.   Adapted from American Society of Addiction Medicine 2020.

Maintenance Pharmacotherapies

The body's neurologic and physiologic adaptations extend beyond the acute withdrawal phase and can account for many behaviors that are hallmarks of AUD (i.e., loss of control over intake, cravings, use despite negative consequences). Pharmacotherapies that aim to reset these chronic adaptations are referred to as medications for alcohol use disorder (MAUD). In targeting the adaptations that characterize addiction, medication-assisted treatment (MAT) supports the changes essential for attaining, and maintaining, recovery from AUD.

Three medications have received FDA approval for treating AUD: naltrexone, disulfiram, and acamprosate. Numerous unapproved (so-called off-label) medications, such as topiramate, gabapentin, and several others, have a growing and compelling evidence base. Topiramate has proven safety and efficacy in treatment of AUD—equal to the FDA-approved MAUD—but trials were conducted after the patent expiration (generic formulation), and therefore FDA approval was not sought. Despite the availability of both FDA-approved and off-label MAUD, these medications remain significantly underutilized (Cohen et al. 2022).

Much of the research supporting the effectiveness of MAT has been conducted with uniform populations, thus excluding individuals with co-occurring medical, social, or psychiatric conditions. This homogeneity limits the generalizability of these medications for treaters working in real-world settings with complex patients, such as those with BPD. Nonetheless, MAT remains a critical option in complex patient popula-

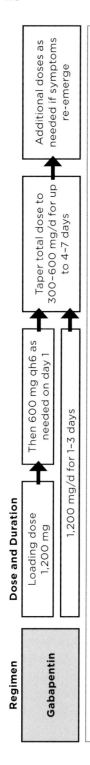
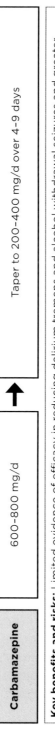
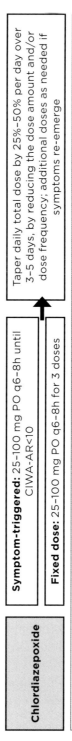

Figure 7–2. Selective outpatient monotherapy alcohol withdrawal regimens for BPD+AUD

tions, especially given the added impacts, risks, and consequences of co-occurring AUD and personality disorders.

In this section, we first review the various pharmacotherapies with a substantial evidence base in the treatment of AUD. This review is followed by a discussion of the use of these pharmacotherapies specifically in individuals with BPD (Gianoli et al. 2012; Kienast et al. 2014; Ralevski et al. 2007). Throughout, we aim to weave in noteworthy clinical considerations specifically pertaining to the principles of GPM in the treatment of BPD.

Pharmacotherapies for AUD all aim to reduce or stop drinking. They can be broken down into two categories: alcohol-sensitizing agents and agents that directly reduce alcohol consumption.

Alcohol-Sensitizing Agents

Alcohol-sensitizing agents disincentivize the consumption of alcohol. They do so by altering the body's processing of alcohol in a way that produces a noxious effect in response to drinking. Therefore, the aim of an alcohol-sensitizing agent is to extinguish the association of pleasure from the ingestion of alcohol by introducing a strong negative association—in other words, to induce the conclusion that "if I drink, I'll get sick." Treatment with an alcohol-sensitizing agents has a particular intuitive appeal, on account of the predictable negative response to alcohol exposure and the consequent 100% abstinence.

Disulfiram (Antabuse) is the only FDA-approved alcohol-sensitizing agent available in the United States. Disulfiram works by irreversibly inhibiting the enzyme aldehyde dehydrogenase, which is responsible for metabolizing acetaldehyde, itself a metabolite of alcohol, into acetic acid. Consequent build-up of acetaldehyde results in the disulfiram-ethanol reaction (DER). DER is characterized by aversive experiences such as flushing, tachycardia, hypotension, nausea, vomiting, shortness of breath, confusion, diaphoresis, and dizziness. More severe symptoms requiring emergency care include cardiac arrythmia and seizures (Segher et al. 2020). Side effects are not common unless patients continue to drink alcohol; however, some patients report headache, fatigue, and dermatitis. Rare fulminant hepatic failure (a medical emergency), optic neuritis, and peripheral neuropathies have been reported. Although rare, these possibilities necessitate periodic liver function testing (monthly during the first 3 months, and quarterly thereafter) and monitoring for vision changes (annual ophthalmologic examinations are recommended) and symptoms of peripheral neuropathy. If neuropathy or optic neuritis emerges, treatment cessation is required.

Disulfiram is usually dosed at 125–500 mg once a day. Because ethanol may be present in a myriad of unexpected foods, beverages, and topical applications, patients need to be warned to be vigilant of possible unintentional ethanol exposures: kombucha and other fermented teas and beverages; "nonalcoholic" beers; vinegar; sauerkraut, kimchi, and other fermented food products; and hand sanitizers (via fume inhalation). Disulfiram is not recommended while pregnant or breastfeeding. Care should be taken when treating individuals with a history of psychotic disorders because of the rare possibility of psychosis exacerbation. Effects of disulfiram may persist for up to 2 weeks after discontinuation.

Disulfiram was approved when FDA efficacy requirements were less rigorous than the current requirements. As a result, despite its widespread use, there is a paucity of large-scale efficacy studies. The one large multicenter trial on disulfiram that is available, conducted in 1986 by the Veterans Administration Cooperative Studies Group, showed that compliance with disulfiram was positively associated with complete abstinence (Fuller et al. 1986). Clinical experience supports these results insofar as disulfiram can be an effective MAT for AUD, provided that the patient takes the medication. As a result, disulfiram appears to be most effective in those individuals whose compliance can be monitored, such as those under court-ordered supervision, or whose family or friends can be enlisted to monitor daily administration (sometimes as part of a formal contract—the so-called sobriety contract of behavioral couples and family therapy) (O'Farrell and Fals-Stewart 2002).

Only two studies have been published of alcohol use outcomes in response to disulfiram treatment for AUD in individuals with BPD. Ralevski et al. (2007) randomly assigned heavy drinking (average of 20 drinks per drinking day) individuals with BPD ($n=68$) or antisocial personality disorder ($n=95$) (DSM-IV criteria [American Psychiatric Association 1994]) into four different treatment arms: naltrexone alone, placebo alone, open-label disulfiram and naltrexone, and open-label disulfiram and placebo. The investigators reported that a diagnosis of either borderline or antisocial personality disorder did not adversely affect alcohol outcomes; nor did those with either personality disorder have a poorer response to medication than individuals without the disorders (Ralevski et al. 2007). The results are difficult to generalize, however, given that the population was recruited from Veterans Administration facilities and were predominantly white (73%) and male (97%). A further limitation is that medication adherence was monitored weekly, not daily.

A case series of eight patients (two male, six female) with AUD and BPD (Mutschler et al. 2010) similarly demonstrated that disulfiram administration demonstrated effectiveness in alcohol drinking outcomes, tolerability, and safety, thereby extending the results reported by Ralevski et al. in a more real-world setting. A strength of the study is that disulfiram was administered three times a week under direct observation by program physicians (Mutschler et al. 2010). It is also worth noting, however, that participants were recruited from a program that first required individuals to complete 3-week inpatient detoxification.

There are safety concerns to keep in mind when considering disulfiram in patients with co-occurring BPD. The effectiveness of disulfiram is largely psychological, in that awareness of DER promotes alcohol as unavailable, which thereby reduces craving and the preoccupation associated with planning to drink. Caution should be used in patients whose impulsivity is severe enough to counter this psychological appreciation, because DER severity increases with the amount of alcohol consumed.

Intentionally "testing" the DER with light alcohol consumption is clinically common and may be discussed in GPM, with a focus on what the patient learned from the test. On its own, the behavior is not a reason to stop disulfiram treatment.

In clinical practice, self-discontinuation of disulfiram is common, limiting its effectiveness. One way to increase medication adherence is through the use of sobriety contracting as part of behavioral couples and family therapy. The contract entrusts a loved one or other trusted person with observing disulfiram daily dosing. The written, signed contract includes detailed terms. One commonly included term is that the trusted support will contact the clinician with concerns if the patient is regularly missing doses. In patients with BPD, this arrangement may inadvertently risk perpetuating the patient's sense of personal ineffectiveness; therefore, care must be taken to ensure that autonomy and agency are explicitly supported.

Medications That Directly Reduce Alcohol Consumption

Whereas alcohol-sensitizing medications disincentivize alcohol intake, other medications directly reduce alcohol consumption. This group of medications alters the experience of ethanol consumption in nonaversive ways, through a variety of mechanisms. For example, medication may decrease the pleasurable experience of drinking, or it may decrease craving. Another effect of medication may be to stabilize neurotransmitter systems that have become disrupted by chronic alcohol use, thereby reducing the vulnerability to relapse. Medications that directly reduce alcohol consumption can be split into three categories: opioidergic medications, acamprosate, and glutamatergic agents.

Opioidergic Medications

The only FDA-approved opioidergic medication for the treatment of AUD is naltrexone. Naltrexone is a strong competitive μ opioid receptor antagonist, often considered the first-line MAT for AUD. Naltrexone is available in oral tablet form, dosed once a day at 50–150 mg. It can also be taken in a 380-mg extended-release injectable preparation (Vivitrol) that is administered every 3–4 weeks. It may initially seem perplexing that blocking opioid receptors would have an impact on alcohol consumption. The mechanism is rooted in the complex neurophysiologic response to alcohol. Upon consumption of alcohol, the brain releases small but physiologically significant amounts of endogenous opioids such as endorphins, which contribute to the pleasurable experience of alcohol consumption. This effect is synergistic with other impacted neurotransmitter systems (serotonin, catecholamines [especially dopamine], and excitatory amino acids [e.g., glutamate]), especially after the first drinks of a drinking episode.

Many studies have supported naltrexone's effectiveness in reducing alcohol consumption, including several comprehensive meta-analyses (Bouza et al. 2004; Jonas et al. 2014; Srisurapanont and Jarusuraisin 2005). Specifically, relative to placebo, naltrexone reduces the likelihood of relapse (especially to heavy drinking), number of drinks per drinking day, and overall percentage of drinking days during treatment. The basis for these effects is that naltrexone potentially decreases craving, reduces alcohol's reinforcing effects, diminishes the experience of intoxication, and reduces the likelihood of continued drinking after a lapse (O'Malley et al. 1996).

Although oral naltrexone is traditionally administered once a day, alternative administration protocols have also shown positive results, such as "targeted administration" in which naltrexone is administered in anticipation of, or in response to, high-risk situations (Heinälä et al. 2001; Kranzler et al. 2003). Common side effects of oral naltrexone include nausea, headache, dizziness, and fatigue. To minimize these side effects, many prescribers initiate treatment at 25 mg for 3–5 days before increasing to the standard 50 mg daily dosing. Rarely, depression and suicidal thinking have been reported with naltrexone initiation, although all controlled trials indicate mood improvement; nonetheless, monitoring for changes in mental status is recommended. Naltrexone may cause hepatic transaminase elevations (increases in aspartate and alanine aminotransferase [AST and ALT]), so baseline and periodic monitoring is recommended (twice a year, or more frequently if changes in medical condition warrant it). Naltrexone is not recommended for use in individuals with liver failure or during pregnancy.

As with disulfiram, ongoing adherence to medication administration is a major challenge to treatment. Extended-release naltrexone presents a useful option for patients who have difficulties adhering to a daily dosing regimen. While a run-in of oral naltrexone is not required for initiating extended-release naltrexone, many treaters opt to initiate oral naltrexone before a trial of extended-release naltrexone (which is administered as a deep gluteal injection) to ensure medication tolerability.

Literature is scant on the effectiveness of naltrexone for the treatment of AUD in individuals with co-occurring BPD. The study by Ralevski et al. (2007), discussed earlier, reported that a diagnosis of either antisocial personality disorder or BPD did not adversely affect alcohol outcomes, nor did those with either personality disorder have a poorer response to medication than people without these disorders.

A small ($N=18$), 8-week, open-label study by Martín-Blanco et al. (2017) examined the effects of nalmefene (an opioid receptor antagonist similar to naltrexone and available for treatment of AUD in some European countries) on alcohol use and BPD symptoms. The authors reported a significant reduction in alcohol consumption, BPD global symptoms, self-injurious behavior, and binge eating. Interestingly, aside from the alcohol-mitigating effects of μ opioid receptor antagonists, the opioid receptor system has been implicated in mediating self-injurious behaviors and other BPD symptoms (Roth et al. 1996; Sonne et al. 1996), which may account for the dual benefits highlighted in the study.

Acamprosate

Acamprosate is an amino acid derivative that enhances the neurotransmission of GABA, which is the main endogenous inhibitory neurotransmitter. Ethanol also strongly enhances GABA transmission, and with repeated exposure to ethanol, endogenous GABA production is reduced and GABA receptors are downregulated. Upon cessation of chronic alcohol use, the balance between inhibitory and excitatory (e.g., glutamate) neurotransmission is tipped in favor of overexcitation because of this downregulation of the inhibitory GABA neurotransmitter system. Unopposed neuroexcitation accounts for many of the symptoms seen in acute alcohol withdrawal syndrome. Even after resolution of acute withdrawal, however, these inhibitory-excitatory systems can remain unbalanced for months to years—a phenomenon known as postacute withdrawal syndrome (PAWS). Patients may experience protracted irritability and dysphoria as well as restlessness, all common interoceptive triggers for substance relapse. Through its effects on GABA neurotransmission, acamprosate appears to mitigate postacute withdrawal symptoms in animal models and in human self-reports, and this mechanism is believed to support abstinence maintenance.

Acamprosate use has a 17% incidence of diarrhea when initiated at full dose (666 mg three times a day). Prescribers often opt to initiate dosing at 333 mg three times a day for 5–7 days before administering the full dose, in a strategy that reduces the probability of side effects. Distinct from naltrexone and disulfiram, acamprosate is renally excreted (unmetabolized), making it an attractive option for patients with significant liver impairment.

It is important to optimize treatment adherence for three-times-a-day dosing. Breakfast, lunch, and dinner mealtime dosing may be a convenient way for patients to remember to take medications, and it is important that acamprosate be taken before meals because of its very poor bioavailability. Prescribers often recommend that, when on the three-times-a-day regimen, the patient pause for a brief recovery ritual or reminder that is personally meaningful. If a patient misses doses regularly, acamprosate will not achieve therapeutic blood levels. There is no target therapy approach with acamprosate; research suggests that patients have optimal outcomes if they have been abstinent for 4–7 days before starting.

Acamprosate gained FDA approval based primarily on the results of three European studies that demonstrated acamprosate's superiority over placebo on two primary outcome measures: continuous abstinence and reduced relapse severity (lower frequency of drinking and less quantity consumed when drinking) (Chick et al. 2003; Kranzler and Gage 2008). Large-scale U.S.-based studies failed to replicate these findings, however, calling into question acamprosate's actual effectiveness as a pharmacotherapy for AUD. In particular, the 11-center placebo-controlled COM-BINE study, which included nearly 1,400 patients, compared naltrexone and acamprosate, alone and in combination, in conjunction with two different behavioral interventions (medical management and an intensive behavioral treatment that included motivational enhancement therapy). Contradicting the European findings, the results of the COMBINE study showed no difference between acamprosate and placebo, either alone or combined with naltrexone (Anton et al. 2006).

Of note, a study that examined the combination of disulfiram and acamprosate demonstrated greater days abstinent when the two medications were combined than when either was administered alone, and also relative to placebo (Besson et al. 1998). The study was not fully randomized. As a consequence of these conflicting effectiveness data in conjunction with its complex dosing regimen, acamprosate is typically considered a second-line MAT for AUD.

To date, no studies have specifically examined acamprosate treatment of AUD in individuals with BPD.

Glutamatergic Agents

Currently, no anticonvulsants are approved by the FDA for the treatment of AUD. Yet the interest in anticonvulsants as a potential treatment for AUD is long-standing and continues to garner research attention. Putatively, the mechanistic rationale for anticonvulsants in MAT is based on their class effects, i.e., glutamate antagonism and GABA agonism. As described earlier, both glutamate antagonism and GABA agonism may counteract the neuroadaptations resulting from chronic ethanol consumption that sustain continued use and perpetuate vulnerability to relapse. A range of anticonvulsants have been studied in the treatment of AUD (including carbamazepine and divalproex), but two of the more commonly studied and prescribed are topiramate and gabapentin.

Topiramate. Topiramate is FDA approved for the treatment of seizure disorder and migraine prophylaxis. Off-label, topiramate is used in the treatment of impulse control disorders, such as binge eating disorder and bulimia nervosa. In patients with AUD, it is used for drinking reduction and recovery maintenance. In maintenance treatment, studies of topiramate have demonstrated superiority relative to placebo across a number of outcomes: number of drinks per drinking day, total drinking days, heavy drinking days, and negative alcohol toxicology screens (Blodgett et al. 2014; Johnson et al. 2003; 2004; 2007; Likhitsathian et al. 2013). Such findings have been especially pronounced in individuals who are actively drinking.

For the treatment of AUD, topiramate is most commonly dosed at 150–300 mg daily. The side effect burden can be significant: paresthesias, tinny taste, fatigue, dizziness, anorexia, nausea, diarrhea, weight loss, and cognitive difficulties (e.g., concentration and word finding, typically occurring at doses ≥300 mg/day). Rarely, increases in suicidal ideation, renal calculi, and acute secondary glaucoma have been reported, and patients with a history of renal calculi or glaucoma are not considered safe candidates for topiramate. For women of childbearing age, it is essential to discuss the risk of teratogenesis and appropriate steps for managing contraception. Many of the side effects can be mitigated by slow dose titration. For example, we recommend starting at 25 mg daily and increasing—in twice-a-day doses—over the course of 8 weeks to a total daily dose of 300 mg. Side effects may prevent many patients from tolerating the full 300-mg dose.

Topiramate is effective in both drinking reduction and abstinence goals, and has the advantage of being safe to initiate in patients who are actively drinking. Topiramate is underutilized because of the titration monitoring requirement and the frequency of side effects; Veteran's Administration guidelines stand out as an exception.

No studies have examined the effectiveness of topiramate specifically in individuals with both AUD and BPD. Interestingly, topiramate was one of three anticonvulsants, alongside lamotrigine and divalproex, identified in a Cochrane review of randomized trials to have beneficial effects on aspects of BPD psychopathology—specifically, anger and impulsive behavioral dyscontrol (Lieb et al. 2010; Nickel et al. 2004; 2005). Thus topiramate may have a role in the treatment of co-occurring AUD and BPD, although further specific research is warranted. A final reason to consider topiramate for BPD+AUD is that 11% of patients will experience a modest weight reduction, which may be appealing if the patient is above ideal body weight.

Gabapentin. Gabapentin is FDA approved for treatment of partial seizures and postherpetic neuralgia. It is also commonly prescribed off-label for the treatment of fibromyalgia, diabetic neuropathy, postsurgical pain and neuropathic pain, anxiety, and insomnia. In patients with AUD, it is prescribed off-label for alcohol withdrawal or recovery maintenance.

Studies of gabapentin in the treatment of AUD (for maintenance) have had mixed results. Some studies demonstrated reduced relapse rates, improved sleep disturbances related to alcohol use, and reduced volume of alcohol consumed when drinking (Brower et al. 2008; Furieri and Nakamura-Palacios 2007; Mariani et al. 2021; Mason et al. 2014; Rentsch et al. 2019). However, a recent meta-analysis of the efficacy of gabapentin for treating AUD found benefit on only one outcome measure relative to placebo: percentage of heavy drinking days (Kranzler et al. 2019).

Positive impacts on AUD have been demonstrated across a wide range of dosing protocols: 300 mg twice a day (Furieri and Nakamura-Palacios 2007), 1,500 mg at bedtime (Brower et al. 2008), 900 mg in the morning and 1,800 mg at bedtime (Mason et al. 2014), and 3,600 mg daily (Mariani et al. 2021). Because the upper limit of gabapentin total daily dosing is 3,600 mg, there is a potentially wide therapeutic window that provides considerable dosing flexibility based on experience.

Gabapentin is generally well tolerated, but common side effects include peripheral edema, nausea, dizziness, fatigue, and ataxia. Rarely, Stevens-Johnson syndrome, suicidality, thought disorder, and respiratory depression have been reported. Of note, gabapentin carries a risk of misuse and addiction, warranting careful monitoring and informed consent to take only as prescribed (Rentsch et al. 2020). Gabapentin is excreted largely unmetabolized, making it (like acamprosate) a viable option for those with significant hepatic impairment. Gabapentin has been shown to be safe even in individuals who are actively drinking (Myrick et al. 2007). Additionally, because of the increasing use of gabapentin in the treatment of alcohol withdrawal, patients who have received gabapentin as part of a detoxification protocol may be more amenable to continuing it for maintenance.

No studies have examined the impact of gabapentin on alcohol use patterns in individuals with AUD+BPD. The evidence for the use of gabapentin in the treatment of BPD without AUD is also scant. One review from Brazil noted positive impacts of gabapentin on aggressiveness and "excitability and turbulent behavior" (Morana and Câmara 2006), and an open-label study from Spain demonstrated global improvements in individuals with BPD as assessed by standardized tools for anxiety, depression, and impulsivity (Peris et al. 2007). It is not prudent to extrapolate from results suggesting gabapentin's effectiveness for AUD and BPD, separately, that gabapentin is therefore useful in treating co-occurring AUD and BPD. More research is warranted.

Others

A host of other medications aiming to treat AUD have been studied, or at least case reports of their use have been published (baclofen and ondansetron). This book is a guide for generalists, so a full accounting of this wide array of medications is beyond our scope, but readers may seek more information in recently published reviews (Burnette et al. 2022).

Choosing Medication

When considering whether to offer medication, and which one, the clinician should give priority to the symptom that causes the greatest impairment. When a BPD symptom causes impairment, treaters can follow the traditional algorithm of GPM—consider medication only on request, or when the illness is severe. When an AUD symptom causes greatest impairment, offer medication proactively.

Of course, some symptoms of BPD can be confused with those of AUD. For example, drinking itself can be indicative of AUD, BPD, or both. Similarly, risky behavior during periods of inebriation, impairment due to drinking, or continuing to drink despite consequences can all be viewed through either an AUD or a BPD lens. First, determine whether AUD or BPD is the best frame for the problem; only then can you choose whether and which medication to offer. To fully explore the provenance of certain symptoms, treaters should create a judgment-free, trusting environment. Such an environment also allows treaters to nurture autonomy, instead of evoking shame or powerlessness.

When drinking indicative of AUD causes concern, treaters should offer medications to reduce intake. Naltrexone is typically offered before acamprosate for the reasons listed earlier.

What is meant by concern? When drinking impacts driving, when it contributes to attempting suicide—either by impairing judgment or by its direct toxic effects—or when medical sequelae of alcohol use are developing. One goal of GPM-AUD is to retain patients in treatment as long as possible, so treaters can offer medication based on their own concern or because patients request it—that is, if a patient identifies drinking as a concern despite the treater thinking otherwise. After a suicide attempt, treaters may offer medication to address not only drinking, but also depression or impulsivity.

When should treaters recommend an alcohol-sensitizing agent? Patients often are not fully adherent with this type of medication because the temptation to skip it and facilitate drinking is too strong. Hence, it should be suggested only when a trusted partner or friend can provide daily supervision of the patient's adherence.

When alcohol use is indicative of BPD rather than AUD, it is better to avoid offering medication. For example, when a breakup leads to intense sadness, crying, and drinking, it is likely that no medication is needed. Instead, treaters can encourage patients to use their social supports and coping skills.

Some situations are complex, with no "right" or "best" approach. One is when patients drink during social interaction and their drinking puts them at risk of being sexually assaulted, either because of the degree of drinking itself or because other risks are present (e.g., a fraternity party or in the company of someone who has previously taken advantage of them). In this situation, we recommend that treaters first encourage nonpharmacologic approaches—coping skills, planning ahead, social support—and also be willing to offer medication as a last resort.

Treaters must be clear that offering medication is based on value, rather than subjective need (the sixth GPM-AUD principle). Value—that is, whether medication "works"—must be defined in a quantifiable way. Clinicians can start by asking patients how they measure value. Simple is best. Counting the number of drinking days, for instance, is a common approach. Tracking a daily rating of cravings, usually on a 1–10 scale, is also useful. When tracking ratings, it is vital to record them prospectively; human memory is too unreliable (Figueiredo et al. 2018) to compare past and current states accurately over more than a few days. Having patients record anything also boosts agency and self-reflection.

Psychological needs that tempt treaters to prescribe could be their own or the patient's. For example, patients and treaters alike can fall into the trap of believing that medication will eliminate distress, taking away the need for the patient to cope with it or tolerate it, even when experience (the treater's or the patient's) has demonstrated that a particular medication, or any medication, is unlikely to help. When this urge arises, the treater can voice the dilemma to the patient and discuss it openly. In the course of this discussion, if both agree that a medication does potentially offer value, the treater may prescribe it. The treater and the patient should then assess the value together within a month's time. (Again, the value of each medication should be reassessed at least quarterly.)

Deprescribing

Medications' value is often short-lived among patients with BPD. Thus, treaters will face situations when medications are ineffective or cease to be effective. The medication should be discontinued—but doing so is anything but simple, of course. Our term for the collaborative process by which treaters discontinue ineffective medications is *deprescribing* (Fineberg et al. 2019).

Deprescribing begins with the offer to prescribe medication: treaters provide an overview of the process of trying medication from beginning to end, including the rationale of continuing only those medications that work. Next, preview how deprescribing will occur and what emotional or behavioral changes can be expected. Patients commonly view deprescribing as a loss, making them reluctant to go along with the idea. To combat that perspective, frame deprescribing as a service for the patient's benefit—freeing them from false hope, from side effects, from delaying a turn to interventions that truly are valuable.

Patients can also be reluctant to stop a medication because they understandably see medication as too powerful. Taking medication makes them feel better, so they fear that taking less will—directly and solely—make them feel worse. If treaters stop or reduce the dose of a medication and patients indeed do experience emotional distress, it's easy for them to view that distress as confirming their initial fear. This attribution, however, is too narrow. It is an example of all-or-nothing thinking applied to medication, which ignores the multitude of reasons that emotions fluctuate: the situation itself, time, bodily states (e.g., fatigue or hunger), and the placebo or nocebo effect, to name a few. This is why previewing expected changes reduces the likelihood that patients will insist on continuing to take a useless medication.

The duration of tapering medication varies based on factors such as trial duration, medication half-life, or likelihood of withdrawal symptoms. In many cases, tapering over 1–2 weeks is sufficient, as with most reuptake inhibitors, dopamine receptor antagonists, and glutamatergic or gabaergic agents. Benzodiazepine receptor agonists and glutamatergic agents are medications that should be tapered slowly to avoid adverse discontinuation syndromes and risk of seizure. When using benzodiazepine receptor agonists, treaters should also consider nonpharmacologic supports to facilitate discontinuation (Soni et al. 2023).

At the appointments after cessation of a medication, check in with the patient about any change in the predefined measurement of value for that medication (e.g., drinking days), as well as about their overall function. Checking in about function reinforces the focus on value, regardless of whether distressing emotions have emerged. If no deterioration occurred, the provider can reassure the patient that that medication is not the right tool to address that particular symptom. Lack of deterioration also reinforces that fear need not be a barrier to deprescribing that is otherwise appropriate. If deterioration did occur, treaters must work with patients to reassess the value of the medication. Re-evaluation is based on what changed, to what degree, and how meaningful that change was. After that analysis, treaters can consider whether the change had meaning despite a quantitative difference. If meaningful benefit was lost, treaters can consider resuming that medication (at the original dose or lower) or trying a new medication.

One way we explain the deprescribing process is as follows:

> We want you to take medication that works, and also not waste your time with medication that doesn't work. It's important to define what "working" means in advance— what medication should do for you. Once we decide that, we'll need to measure the value of the medication as we go. If we find that one of your medications isn't helping, we'll stop it, gradually if necessary. When we stop medication, if we're right that it wasn't helping, you won't notice a thing. It's like if you subtract zero; ten minus zero is still ten.
>
> Even so, people can have a psychological reaction to knowing that we are changing medication, a placebo effect. Because of that psychological reaction, emotional ups and downs are common as we reduce the dose. Sometimes people worry that the emotional ups and downs are a sign that we made a bad decision, that reducing the medication makes them worse, but most often that's not the case. We'll want to pay attention to the overall pattern of your [primary symptom] with and without medication, not just the fluctuations at one moment. And, if we discover that the medication is more valuable than we thought, it's always possible to go back on it.

Deprescribing can be challenging when patients have been on several medications for a while. In such cases, patients cannot be expected to remember how effective, or not, a medication has been. Moreover, patients are rarely taught the harms of polypharmacy. In other cases, removing ineffective medications is difficult because patients have attached meaning or value to them that is subjective and cannot be substantiated. For example, patients may believe that treatment is hopeless if a certain medication doesn't work for them. Patients taking several medications are often highly symptomatic or unstable emotionally, so even when patients are willing to stop taking medication, repeated crises may exhaust all of the clinical attention, leaving treaters without sufficient time or inclination to remove medication and making them think they will delay deprescribing until the situation is somehow better.

Repeated crises are unlikely to remit spontaneously, however, and they serve as a clear indication that the current medications offer little to no benefit. Furthermore, when crises repeat frequently, the patient is experiencing too little agency and autonomy. Insufficient agency or autonomy can lead to excess focus on external factors, including medication, that seem to control the patient's experience. Therefore, especially amid crises, treaters should prioritize stopping medications that do not provide demonstrable value.

Conclusion

BPD and AUD co-occur often. When they do, outcomes are worse. The vulnerability of this population makes a structured approach all the more valuable. GPM-AUD espouses eight principles to provide that structure. Treaters should address both disorders simultaneously, building a framework that integrates medical and 12-step models. Treaters should prioritize safety and retention. Treating AUD actively using standard-of-care approaches is essential for mitigating suicide risk, symptomatic severity, and clinical complexity for individuals with BPD. We recommend negotiating for behavior change, while always encouraging autonomy. Medication targeting AUD can be offered proactively. If medication adds value, it can be continued, while still avoiding unnecessary polypharmacy.

Medications for AUD work in a variety of ways. When considering medication, treaters must first determine what the most impairing symptom is, and whether that symptom can be attributed to AUD or BPD. Treaters should also be wary of the temptation to use medication to address psychological needs, be they their own or the patient's. Nevertheless, retaining patients in treatment is paramount, so medications can be offered or continued even when the treater is skeptical of their value. Doing so may also serve to nurture and honor patients' autonomy.

Once treaters decide to offer medication, they should plant the seeds of deprescribing from the outset—discussing the goal of medication use, how to measure progress toward that goal, and the anticipated duration of use. When a symptom of AUD causes considerable impairment, several medications are available, three of which are currently approved by the FDA. These agents can either sensitize patients to the effects of alcohol (disulfiram) or reduce drinking (naltrexone and acamprosate). Other off-label options, such as topiramate and gabapentin, serve to reduce drinking. Prescribing should always be done in tandem with nonpharmacologic supports or interventions.

8

Multimodal Treatments

Edward Patzelt, Ph.D.
Stephen Conway, M.D.
Lois W. Choi-Kain, M.D., M.Ed.

Human beings have an inherent desire to form and maintain relationships. A social network helps individuals manage stress and self-regulate, and ultimately it improves both mental and physical health (Baumeister and Leary 1995; Baumeister et al. 2005; Cohen 2004; Cohen and Wills 1985). A robust social network can serve to buffer the stress-sensitive vulnerabilities of individuals with borderline personality disorder plus alcohol use disorder (BPD+AUD), yet patients with BPD typically have reduced social support: they tend toward smaller support networks with greater interpersonal conflict and less social integration (Beeney et al. 2018; Lazarus et al. 2016). Social networks often shrink over time in individuals with AUD, as binge drinking creates social and occupational losses. Social isolation is a risk for relapse in AUD, and the drinking behaviors of one's social network significantly influence alcohol use (Mowbray et al. 2014; Stout et al. 2012; Zywiak et al. 2002).

In good psychiatric management of BPD and AUD (GPM-AUD), we use multimodal clinical resources to expand the treatment team and strengthen the social network for individuals with BPD and alcohol use problems. Patients with BPD+AUD benefit from tailored guidance in forming a social network that promotes abstinence and recovery (Brooks et al. 2017; Litt et al. 2009). GPM-AUD promotes multimodal treatment

135

(groups, family involvement, case management), a structured, pragmatic, and collaborative approach that incorporates multiple treatment options. Multimodal treatment models the formation of an effective social network and social safety net for the patient. This holistic approach addresses pertinent medical and psychosocial factors, improves patient outcomes, reduces treatment-interfering behaviors, and increases treatment retention. Quality of life is improved for both the patient and family members, and clinician burnout is decreased.

Selecting Other Modalities and Establishing the Treatment Frame

Several modalities can be considered when constructing a treatment plan for patients with BPD + AUD (Table 8–1). Patients with BPD commonly engage in some degree of multimodal treatment: 75% see a mental health professional, such as a physician, therapist, or counselor, and 63% are prescribed medication (Tomko et al. 2014). Compared with major depressive disorder and other personality disorders, patients with BPD more commonly utilize individual and group therapy (but not family/couples psychotherapy or mutual-help groups) (Bender et al. 2001). For individuals seeking abstinence from alcohol and drug use problems, mutual-help organizations (MHOs) (e.g., Alcoholics Anonymous and other 12-step programs, SMART Recovery) are most commonly utilized (45%), followed by professional treatment (outpatient, inpatient, residential, or detoxification services) (28%), recovery support services defined as faith-based or community center services (22%), and medication (9%) (Kelly et al. 2017). For patients with both disorders, it is important to provide psychoeducation about the numerous options to promote informed decisions when establishing a tailored treatment plan.

There are several factors to consider when selecting another modality, such as the severity of each disorder, patient preference, motivation to change, and current life stability (e.g., housing, transportation, finances). A common multimodal treatment for BPD + AUD is composed of a prescriber/psychiatrist (or primary care provider) and an individual therapist plus mutual-help group, with or without family interventions. Accessibility and cost may limit the treatment planning, and care teams can meet these challenges in creative ways by incorporating virtual care services and community resources freely available to the patient, reinforcing the central aim to increase social integration. At minimum, the prescriber/psychiatrist or primary care provider will assume the role of

Table 8-1. **Complementary functions of different modalities**

Modality	Functions
Substance counseling/therapy	Provide alcohol counseling, motivational interviewing, time-limited protocols
Individual psychotherapy	Help clarify and validate a sense of self; help learn to think first and recognize cause-and-effect patterns; offer corrective experiences within the therapeutic alliance
Care management	Advise on activities of daily living, work and family initiatives, budget, diet, etc.
Medication management	Provide outpatient withdrawal management; prescribe medications (moderate to severe AUD or binge drinking; other substance use disorders, such as smoking cessation; other mental health disorders; when necessary, targeted symptom relief of BPD crises); address co-occurring medical issues related to alcohol and other substance use; when medically necessary, initiate referral to higher levels of care
Group therapy (see Table 8–3)	Work on social skills, self-awareness, self-disclosure, empathy, and affect tolerance; promote self-efficacy through mutual peer support
Mutual-help groups (see Table 8–4)	Provide social support, encourage sharing/self-disclosure, offer skills training to promote abstinence
Family interventions (education and skills training for family to support treatment) (see Tables 8–10 and 8–11)	Provide psychoeducation on decreasing situation stress, increasing support, improving quality of life for family members

Note. AUD = alcohol use disorder; BPD = borderline personality disorder.
Source. Adapted from Gunderson and Links 2014.

both psychopharmacologist (who will also address medical concerns related to alcohol use) and GPM-informed therapist in combination with the patient's active participation in a mutual-help group (as these groups are widely available, accessible, and free). For patients with difficulty managing their basic needs (shelter, food, finances, transportation, child care, etc.), care management is a priority to establish a safe treatment frame for therapeutic interventions; such resources are coordinated by regionally available social services or by referral within the patient's health care plan.

A well-structured treatment establishes clear roles among the treatment team members and promotes open communication with the patient's full consent (Table 8–2).

Common Problems With Setting the Treatment Frame

Your Patient Devalues the Other Treater

A core strategy of multimodal treatment is to neither validate nor object to complaints about another treater. This encourages the patient to lean in and work through conflicts and complaints in relationships. When a patient has a complaint regarding one of their treaters, express concern and explore what underlies the patient's hostile feelings. It is important that the patient directly address the complaint with the treater, as this can serve as a corrective experience when that treater does not respond by withdrawing or becoming angry. In cases where the patient refuses to talk to the other treater, it may be best to pursue a group meeting. Sometimes this must be presented as nonnegotiable, especially if the qualm is with the primary treater. Overall, acquiescing to a patient's refusal to address complaints to the other therapist is never helpful, as it reinforces splitting within social networks.

Your Cotreater Is Not Adhering to the Frame

Successful treatment involves open communication among team members; however, the demands within health care delivery systems complicate optimal care team communications and meetings. As long as team members maintain the framework regarding roles and communicate promptly about safety concerns (including safety concerns related to drinking) and recurrent treatment nonadherence, in many cases this is sufficient. If the other treater is noncommunicative and their interventions are harmful, then this indicates a lapse in the treatment framework, and a consultation may be helpful. If the treatment structure is failing, the lead GPM provider must review it with the patient to determine how best to support them; sometimes less treatment is more stabilizing for the patient.

Table 8–2. Framework for multimodal treatments for patients with BPD + AUD

Establish clear roles: determine which treater will manage safety, monitor drinking behavior, address alcohol-related medical concerns (e.g., treat alcohol withdrawal first; assess hepatic dysfunction), provide psycho-education about BPD + AUD and treatment as well as medical consequences of alcohol use, evaluate progress toward goals, and authorize treatment changes

Treaters communicate at their discretion—but always about safety (including safety concerns related to drinking) and recurrent nonadherence to the treatment plan

Treaters need to understand and respect each other's complementary roles

Note. AUD = alcohol use disorder; BPD = borderline personality disorder.
Source. Adapted from Gunderson and Links 2014.

Your Cotreater Thinks You Must Address BPD (or AUD) First in the Treatment Plan

A treatment plan must be agreed on by all members of the treatment team. GPM-AUD promotes integrated care approaches as optimal, with medical safety prioritized in the treatment plan. This may mean that inpatient care needs to precede outpatient care if the patient requires AUD withdrawal management or containment of suicide risk, but otherwise therapeutic stabilization addresses all mental disorders simultaneously. An open discussion of care team concerns helps to establish clarity of team roles and responsibilities.

Group Therapy

Group therapy has the potential to provide powerful corrective relational experiences. At the same time, many patients with BPD + AUD resist attending or participating in groups out of concern about what other group members will think of them, because they feel shame related to their drinking, or in some cases, because they don't want to share attention. Clinicians can encourage group attendance to decrease avoidance; it may even be a requirement for participation in individual psychotherapy.

Group therapy offers the opportunity for social learning in a safe environment. Individuals can develop the capacity to listen, share, and engage collaboratively with others while gaining self-awareness and self-understanding. It is a space where individuals relate experiences and feelings, increase self-acknowledgment of problems, and learn that others struggle with similar problems and have different coping mechanisms. Patients often report that the most powerful information or feedback came from a peer. Group members are in different stages of BPD and AUD recovery, so those earlier in the process may become more hopeful as they witness others stably established in recovery. Challenges in navigating interpersonal dynamics are certain to arise as BPD symptoms emerge in group interactions. These challenges offer an opportunity to learn in the moment as well as provide experiences to work through with the individual therapist.

As mentioned earlier in "Selecting Other Modalities and Establishing the Treatment Frame," mutual-help groups, such as 12-step programs and SMART Recovery, are widely available, accessible, and free. There are several other evidence-based group therapy options to consider, such as clinician-facilitated AUD or BPD treatment groups and BPD+AUD integrated group therapies such as Women's Recovery Group (Greenfield et al. 2014) (Table 8–3). Selection of a group should be collaborative, considering the patient's preferences and the recommendation of the clinician. The clinician must consider the severity of BPD and AUD symptoms and determine whether a more structured or clinician-led group may be suitable. If the patient is motivated, a skills-training group is beneficial.

Mutual-Help Groups

A wide range of mutual-help groups are available. Women for Sobriety, LifeRing, SMART Recovery, and Alcoholics Anonymous are community-led peer groups conferring similar benefits in reduction of alcohol use (Zemore et al. 2018). Alcoholics Anonymous is the most widely available option for patients (Kelly 2022), with the strongest empirical support (Kelly et al. 2020).

Alcoholics Anonymous

Alcoholics Anonymous (AA) is an efficacious, cost-effective, and widely available option as an additional therapeutic modality for BPD+AUD patients (Kelly 2022). Worldwide, AA has more than 2 million members in 180 countries and hundreds of thousands of meetings in person, by phone or internet, and in most languages (www.aa.org). Active AA involvement consistently predicts drinking outcomes up to 10 years past the onset of abstinence (Kelly et al. 2020; Pagano et al. 2013; Witbrodt et

Table 8–3. Hierarchy of group therapies for patients with BPD+AUD[a]

Type of group	Emphasis
Mutual-help groups (12-step programs, SMART Recovery, Recovery Dharma, Dual Recovery Anonymous, Refuge Recovery, Women for Sobriety)	Support, social networking, clarity, simplicity, promote abstinence; see Table 8–4 for further descriptions
Clinical self-assessment and relapse prevention groups	Support, self-disclosure, listening, activities of daily living
Skills building (DBT skills are the preeminent example)	Didactic, self-regulatory skills are prioritized to allow secondary social skills development
Interpersonal (MBT)	Closeness, trust

Note. AUD=alcohol use disorder; BPD=borderline personality disorder; DBT=dialectical behavior therapy; MBT=mentalization-based therapy; SMART=Self-Management and Recovery Training.
[a]In terms of availability, costs, and capability of patients.
Source. Adapted from Gunderson and Links 2014.

Table 8–4. Mutual-help organizations

Group name	Brief description
Alcoholics Anonymous	12-step program, spiritually based (higher power), peer-led, abstinence-based
SMART Recovery	Influenced by CBT, MET, and MI; secular, peer-led, abstinence-based
Recovery Dharma	Based on Buddhist teachings, peer-led, abstinence-based
Women for Sobriety	13 affirmations aimed at changing self-image and world view; secular, women-only, peer-led, abstinence-based
Dual Recovery Anonymous	12-step program, spiritually based, peer-led, abstinence-based, dual diagnosis (psychiatric and substance use disorder)
Refuge Recovery	Based on Buddhist teachings, peer-led, abstinence-based

Note. CBT=cognitive-behavioral therapy; MET=motivational enhancement therapy; MI=motivational interviewing; SMART=Self-Management and Recovery Training.

al. 2014). Although BPD+AUD patients often resist AA due to fluctuations in motivation, ambivalence about alcohol use, changes in the therapeutic alliance, and overall symptom severity, the GPM-AUD clinician
can have significant influence on the patient's AA involvement (Manning
et al. 2012). Therefore, this portion of the chapter is aimed at helping the
treater successfully facilitate the patient's involvement with AA.

***12-Step Facilitation and Alcoholics Anonymous: Efficacy and Mech-
anisms of Change.***   12-Step facilitation (TSF) is a treatment protocol
for therapists to facilitate patient AA involvement (Nowinski and Baker
1992). TSF and AA have demonstrated considerable success in absti-
nence-related outcomes such as drinking intensity, percentage of days
abstinent, alcohol addiction severity, and alcohol-related consequences
(Kelly et al. 2020). TSF/AA outperforms other empirically supported
treatments (e.g., cognitive-behavioral therapy, motivational enhancement therapy) in achieving long-term abstinence, AUD remission within
12 months, and AUD remission up to 3 years after the end of treatment.
Furthermore, TSF/AA is cost-effective, providing a health care cost sav-
ings of $10,000 per patient over 2 years. Manualized TSF provides a
greater benefit than unstructured approaches, and the key ingredient of
TSF is its ability to successfully facilitate AA involvement.

The ways in which AA confers benefit are rooted in social, cognitive,
affect, and behavioral mechanisms. They include changes in social networks, social abstinence, and self-efficacy (i.e., the ability to cope in social situations without alcohol use) and improvements in recovery
motivation, impulsivity, craving, coping skills, negative affect, and spirituality (Kelly 2022). Women benefit most from an increased ability to
cope with negative affect without alcohol use, as well as reductions in depression. Comparatively, men benefit most from increased confidence in
their ability to cope in the presence of alcohol during high-risk social situations, as well as social network shifts toward recovery-oriented peers.
Similarly, young adults benefit most through exclusion of alcohol/drug-
using individuals from their social network. Together, these findings
suggest that consideration should be given to the demographic characteristics of the BPD+AUD patient when facilitating AA involvement.

Alcoholics Anonymous: A Preponderance of Social Support.   Social
support consistently predicts outcomes in BPD (Beeney et al. 2018; Howard and Cheavens 2023; Ingkachotivanich et al. 2022; Thadani et al. 2022;
Zielinski and Veilleux 2014) and AUD (Kaskutas et al. 2002; Kelly and

Hoeppner 2013; Witbrodt and Kaskutas 2005). Much like group therapy, AA provides a safe environment for learning. Patients are exposed to dozens, if not hundreds, of different narratives. This can elicit deep identification with the problems of alcohol use. Moreover, the predominance of successful recovery in AA generates a community of people actively addressing problems with alcohol use, identity, and relationships. Along with this, AA has several advantages for the GPM-AUD clinician. AA is available throughout the day—on virtual platforms, 24 hours per day— allowing patients to address emotional stress in vivo through social support. Agency and commitment develop through choosing AA meetings, selecting a sponsor, and working through the 12 steps of recovery with a sponsor. A sponsor is independent of the care team and does not typically share information with the team, instead providing confidential coaching to assist a patient with achieving sobriety goals.

Alcoholics Anonymous Facilitation: Meetings, Sponsorship, Working the 12 Steps, Spirituality, and Service. It can be difficult to know where to start with the BPD + AUD patient. Most patients will have been exposed to AA (Manning et al. 2012); a common retort is that "AA does not work." This sentiment is also common for AA-naive patients and can be overcome by dispelling common myths about AA (Table 8–5). Regardless of past involvement, future AA involvement predicts later abstinence (Tonigan et al. 2017). Simple directives to attend AA, or get a sponsor, are unlikely to work. Therefore, using motivational techniques throughout treatment will increase successful AA facilitation (Vederhus et al. 2014).

When patient motivation wanes, an understandably common therapeutic mistake is to abandon AA facilitation. However, there is a dose-dependent response between AA facilitation and later attendance (Pfund et al. 2021), such that persistence will increase AA involvement. On a practical level, AA facilitation requires consistent assessment and intervention around key aspects of AA involvement (see Table 8–6, "Session Checklist" for questions to discuss with patients). It is highly recommended that persons new to AA be referred initially to a beginner's meeting, where the facilitator explains how AA works and how to get started in the program.

Once they are engaged in AA, the most persistent challenge with BPD + AUD patients is underinvolvement. Despite the best intentions of both treater and patient, the goal of AA involvement can be neatly evaded, and the evasion becomes apparent only after significant alcohol

Table 8–5.   Myths About Alcoholics Anonymous

Myth	Truth
"AA is a religious program."	AA is a spiritual program about seeking a connection with something bigger than yourself.
"Everyone in AA is old."	Most cities have young people's meetings.
"AA is a cult."	AA welcomes everyone having the desire to improve problems with alcohol use, but AA does not recruit members.
"AA is only for people who use alcohol."	AA will welcome anyone with a desire to stop using substances, but the focus is on alcohol cessation.
"I have to identify as an alcoholic to be in AA."	The only requirement for membership is that the person has a desire to stop drinking (or using substances).
"AA won't help with my anxiety or depression."	AA only promotes sobriety, but working toward sobriety within a fellowship reduces anxiety and depression and increases psychological well-being.

use consequences. Amid the chaos of family problems, life-threatening behaviors, and alcohol use, the idea of finding a home group (the specific meeting a person commits to attend to facilitate development of a peer recovery network), getting a sponsor, or working the 12 steps might feel trivial to both the patient and the treater. This is understandable and can be validated with the patient. Returning to the original goals of the treatment can help reorient the patient toward the need to focus on AA involvement.

It is important to work with the patient to identify roadblocks. Look for interpersonal events that may have triggered interpersonal hypersensitivity leading to underinvolvement. Rejection sensitivity (Zielinski and Veilleux 2014), negative first impressions (Hepp et al. 2021), sponsorship alliance (Kelly et al. 2016a, 2016b), and perceived AA group cohesion (Kuerbis and Tonigan 2018) can influence AA involvement. Early in treatment, the patient may have vague awareness of these triggers. More commonly, they will say that their sponsor does not understand them, they cannot find a good meeting, or they tried AA and it did not work. Do not be dissuaded. Persist in examining the patient's involvement. Understanding underinvolvement often requires a dynamic deconstructive psychotherapy analysis or chain analysis. Very few patients will report overall dissatisfaction with AA if they are actively involved with a home group and a sponsor and progressing through the 12 steps.

Table 8–6. Session checklist for AA facilitation

Area of interest	Questions
Overall attitude toward AA	Are you finding AA to be helpful? Why or why not? (assess BPD symptoms such as splitting, interpersonal hypersensitivity, and AUD)
AA meetings	What meetings are you attending/have you attended? How did you experience the meetings?
Sponsorship	Have you identified someone to be your sponsor? How often have you spoken with your sponsor? How do you feel toward your sponsor? (assess the quality of the relationship)
Step work and spirituality (once sponsor relationship is established, the sponsor will guide this)	What step are you working on with your sponsor? What concerns/issues have you encountered while working the steps? Are you involved in any service work? If so, what? If not, what might be getting in the way?

Note. AA = Alcoholics Anonymous; AUD = alcohol use disorder; BPD = borderline personality disorder.

Alcoholics Anonymous Meetings. The goal is to help the patient find an AA home group (more details about home groups are found later in this chapter, "The Therapeutic Environment of Home Groups"). This is a meeting, or meeting location, that they attend at least weekly, sometimes daily. Consistent attendance supports accountability and builds a safety net. Essentially, relationships develop with home group members who will ask the patient about nonattendance, sponsorship, and step progress. In moments of dire need (e.g., alcohol craving), recovery peers are available for support and provide a social support network. Hold the patient accountable to finding a home group; look up meetings, predict interpersonal obstacles, and review the patient's experience of the meetings during sessions. With your patient, collaboratively anticipate challenges of interpersonal hypersensitivity (e.g., perceived hostility, rejection sensitivity, splitting). This helps the patient tolerate the discomfort of building relationships with new people and inoculates them against early AA dropout.

There are thousands of online and in-person AA meetings with a myriad of demographics, including women's, men's, young people's, and LGBTQ+ meetings. Alongside demographics, meetings vary widely in their focus, such as review of specific steps, reading from AA literature, speaker meetings (e.g., a member shares their recovery experiences), or open sharing (all group members discuss current recovery challenges and experiences). Despite this variety, patients may report they cannot find a good meeting. Pause to consider issues of ambivalence, motivation, shame, and interpersonal vulnerabilities. Meetings vary in size; patients who prefer smaller-sized groups can try early morning meetings, which tend to be smaller and have a greater number of members in sobriety maintenance than meetings later in the day.

Sponsorship. Help the patient find a sponsor and sustain the relationship. Having a strong sponsorship alliance is associated with AA involvement, step work completion, and abstinence (Gomes and Hart 2009; Kelly et al. 2016a, 2016b; Subbaraman et al. 2011; Tonigan and Rice 2010). Initially, the prospect of trusting a sponsor is daunting (Fonagy et al. 2015a), and a helpful strategy is for the patient to request a "temporary sponsor," which allows the pair to assess whether the relationship is a good fit before determining maintenance sponsorship. Early sponsorship affiliation is critical and predicts later abstinence (Tonigan and Rice 2010). Patients may report prior sponsorship as unsuccessful. Collaboratively think through these experiences. Lack of regular contact, incomplete 12-step work, and perceived hostility may drive negative impressions of prior sponsorship. With your patient, consider the benefits of sponsorship, such as a history of shared problems with alcohol use, access to immediate support, and a sponsor's success in recovery. Ask them who they identify with in the meetings, and why. Direct them toward sponsors that have the life they want. Encourage them to speak with fellow AA members about challenges with finding a sponsor. When successful, anticipate significant reliance on sponsorship, especially early in GPM treatment and AA involvement.

After the patient has a sponsor, sustaining engagement in the program is key and predicts later abstinence (Witbrodt et al. 2012). Continuously assess splitting. BPD+AUD patients may steer toward enmeshment, idealize the sponsor, and seek constant sponsor contact. They may also be defensive and rejecting, feeling slighted when their sponsor suggests change. Assess regularity of contact and sponsorship alliance. Inability to meet a sponsor's expectations (e.g., regular contact, step work) can lead to avoidance, and may appear as devaluation. Differentiate between the need for a change in sponsor and AA underinvolvement.

Effective sponsors will insist on progress through the 12 steps via extensive reading and writing from the AA basic text, colloquially the Big

Book (Gomes and Hart 2009). The step work might raise ambivalence about change, shame, and crises of identity. Validate these difficulties and encourage the patient to discuss challenges with the sponsor. Often, a conversation with the sponsor is a corrective experience, highlighting how the sponsor navigated similar struggles and their continued intention to help the BPD+AUD patient. Moreover, the joint reflection between sponsor and sponsee may begin challenging insecure attachment styles (Agrawal et al. 2004; Vungkhanching et al. 2004) and increase reflective functioning (Jordan 2019).

Working the 12 Steps. Encourage the patient to progress in working the 12 steps. Step work reduces depression and cravings (Wiebe et al. 2018), while increasing abstinence (Gomes and Hart 2009; Greenfield and Tonigan 2013; Magill et al. 2015). A common obstacle is that the patient reports progress in the steps without having a sponsor. Intellectualizing, purported understanding, and rationalizing all contribute to lack of step progress. Avoidance is understandable, as the 12 steps are a deeply involved process (see Table 8–7 for an overview of the 12 steps) and include admission of the inability to control drinking, surrender of omnipotence, self-examination, relationship repair, and daily spiritual practices. Resistance is natural and can be validated (see Table 8–8 for common problems). Step work ought to proceed slowly to achieve mastery at each step before moving to the next step, and it will take months to years for completion, as it is not uncommon for relapse episodes to disrupt progress; many members move through the 12 steps repeatedly. This can make assessment of progress confusing. Focus on highlighting the sponsor's assessment of progress. This reduces the burden on the treater and places the need for forward progress with the patient. When stuck, turn the patient toward AA members for help. Asking for help increases agency and improves social problem-solving skills.

Spirituality. Spirituality is an experiential and emotional process associated with feelings of hope, love, connection, inner peace, comfort, and support (Anandarajah and Hight 2001). Because of spirituality's association with the etiology, diagnosis, and treatment of psychopathology, the World Health Organization now recommends its direct integration throughout treatment (Moreira-Almeida et al. 2016). Indeed, BPD is associated with lower levels of spirituality compared with the general public (Sansone et al. 2012); increases in spirituality and spiritual practices predict beneficial alcohol use outcomes (Kelly et al. 2011; Krentzman et

Table 8–7.　Overview of the Alcoholics Anonymous 12 steps and 12-step process

Step	Virtues	Purpose	Possible outcomes
1. Admitted we were powerless over alcohol—that our lives had become unmanageable.	Honesty	Awareness and acceptance of inability to control drinking	Sense of identification with other members or decreased sense of aloneness
2. Came to believe that a power greater than ourselves could restore us to sanity.	Hope	Instill a belief that one can recover with help from a higher power	Increased sense of trust; decreased sense of omnipotence
3. Made a decision to turn our will and our lives over to the care of [higher power].	Faith	Commitment to the rest of the steps and seeking direction from a higher power for living	Decreased reliance on maladaptive thinking patterns; sense of freedom; anxiety about step 4
4. Made a searching and fearless moral inventory of ourselves.	Courage	Identify ways in which maladaptive responses to emotions have led to drinking and negative consequences in relationships	Emotional exposure to shame; appreciate personal patterns of negative emotions and behaviors
5. Admitted to [higher power], to ourselves, and to another human being the exact nature of our wrongs.	Integrity	Remove shame; corrective experience of being accepted; internalize sense of responsibility	Self-acceptance; increased sense of belonging and connectedness; accountability
6. Were entirely ready to have [higher power] remove all these defects of character.	Willingness	Readiness to actually change these components of oneself	Openness (willing and ready) to new ideas
7. Humbly asked [higher power] to remove our shortcomings.	Humility	Acknowledge imperfections and ask for help	Increased sense of agency in the process of asking for help

Table 8–7. Overview of the Alcoholics Anonymous 12 steps and 12-step process (*continued*)

Step	Virtues	Purpose	Possible outcomes
8. Made a list of all persons we had harmed, and became willing to make amends to them all.	Love	Recognize how personal shortcomings have affected others and openness to repair relationships	Increased desire to repair relationships; fear about the response of others
9. Made direct amends to such people wherever possible, except when to do so would injure them or others.	Discipline	Take accountability for their behavior in the relationship; repair prior harms	Learn how to have equal relationships with people; less avoidance of interpersonal challenges
10. Continued to take personal inventory and when we were wrong promptly admitted it.	Patience/ perseverance	Sustained effort to watch for dishonesty, anxiety, anger, self-focused attention; maintain personal integrity and relationships through quick repair	Personality change; increased sense of integration and coherence
11. Sought through prayer and meditation to improve conscious contact with [higher power], praying only for knowledge of [higher power's] will for us and the power to carry that out.	Awareness	Development and maintenance of an inner compass and morality to guide decision-making	A sense of connectedness to other people and broader humanity; more present
12 After a spiritual awakening as the result of these steps, we tried to carry this message to alcoholics, and to practice these principles in all our affairs.	Service	Acknowledgement of significant personality change, commitment to sharing the hope of the 12-step process and living the principles outlined in the previous steps	More focused on the needs of others

Source. 12 Steps text from Alcoholics Anonymous 2002.

Table 8–8. Common problems patients encounter in AA

Steps (corresponding stage of change)	Common problems with AA engagement	Common problems with the step work	GPM principles in step work
1–3 (program commitment steps/surrender)	Underinvolvement: not calling sponsor; not sharing honestly with sponsor and home group; not consistently attending home group	Patient does not believe AA can help; believes they can control their drinking; has discomfort with spirituality of program	Psychoeducation; fosters accountability; change is expected
4–9 (action steps)	Not talking about difficulty with step work (e.g., fourth step) with sponsor and in meetings (pretend mode); not calling sponsor; reduction in meeting attendance	Patient stalls on fourth step writing; keeps a secret in fifth step; stalls on eighth step list; stalls on ninth step amends	Fosters accountability; focus on life outside treatment; be active, not reactive
10–12 (maintenance steps)	Reduction in meeting attendance (e.g., home group); not doing service work (e.g., sponsoring, meeting jobs)	Does not have daily meditation and prayer	Fosters accountability; learning to think first

Note. AA = Alcoholics Anonymous; GPM = good psychiatric management.

al. 2017; Tonigan et al. 2013; Wnuk 2021). Individuals often report that spirituality (but not religiosity) aids in their recovery (Kelly and Eddie 2020), and a belief in a higher power reduces both cravings and depression (Galanter et al. 2020). Moreover, spirituality increases well-being, with increases in hope predicting abstinence and AA involvement (Wnuk 2015; 2017; 2021; 2022).

Despite these advantages, patients often struggle with spirituality and the concept of a higher power. Surrender and powerlessness are direct challenges to the desire for omnipotence (McGlashan 1983; Zanarini et al. 2009b). Validate this desire, inquire about its utility, and examine its consequences. Atheistic or agnostic views are no barrier to AA involvement, as Secular AA options exist (https://www.aasecular.org/).

Be mindful of the patient's progress in working the 12 steps. Patients will use objections to spirituality as reason to resist finding a sponsor and starting step work. This may reflect ambivalence about change. Use of motivational interviewing, treatment goals, and the therapeutic frame can help the patient overcome these initial hurdles. Ambivalence about spirituality often arises during step 3 (turn will and lives over to higher power) and can be driven by fear about completion of step 4 (make searching and fearless moral inventory). Ask the patient how AA members deal with struggles of spirituality. Direct them toward discussions with AA members and their sponsor. The AA community is well versed in overcoming challenges with spirituality. Like overcoming problems of identity, moving through this obstacle is slow. During sessions, discussions of spirituality and a higher power can be therapeutically appropriate; however, be wary of intellectualization and rationalization. Broadly, redirection toward reliance on the AA fellowship and sponsorship is a potent intervention.

A Note on Service Work. Service work in AA predicts positive AUD outcomes (Pagano et al. 2013; Zemore and Kaskutas 2004; 2008). Indeed, helping others is touted by AA members as prophylactic and a remedy for rumination. BPD+AUD patients struggle deeply with rumination, putting them at risk for affective instability (Richman Czégel et al. 2022) and alcohol use (Devynck et al. 2019). Helping others, greeting members before AA meetings, pouring coffee, and calling other AA members increases self-efficacy. Encourage AA service work. Objections regarding time restrictions indicate ambivalence about AA involvement. Persist in recommending service to others. This strengthens the social network.

Over time, service work becomes a central part of recovery and translates to broader community involvement (Zemore and Kaskutas 2004).

Common Problems in AA

Interpersonal hypersensitivity can be a major barrier to AA integration. Enmeshment and estrangement are both problematic. When threatened, alone, or despairing, patients turn to isolation. It may be unrelated to AA or could also be the consequence of rejection sensitivity and perceived hostility. Begin with assessment. Use techniques such as chain analysis to uncover what prompted the decompensation. It could be a relapse, fight with a partner, or comment from an AA member. Once the cause is discovered, create a holding environment for this experience and collaboratively reconsider involvement with AA. If the patient resists this discussion, return to validation. Resistance suggests that the patient does not feel connected or contained enough to consider returning to AA.

Enmeshment can lead to catastrophic exits from AA. The warmth and acceptance common to AA meetings can be a powerful motivator for enmeshment. Patients often find their new "favorite person" upon entry to AA. This could be a friend, group of friends, or romantic interest. Friends can be beneficial when they are actively involved in AA. Early in treatment, romantic interests threaten sobriety and recovery, and AA advises against romantic relationships during the first year of sobriety. Balance skepticism with support. Dissuading the patient from romantic pursuits is unlikely to work, but it may be helpful to articulate AA's position on this, which is rooted in the observation that romantic relationships distract the individual from prioritizing sobriety efforts and self-care. Focus on the therapeutic alliance and emotional containment while expressing concerns about enmeshment.

Patient Went in the Past, But Won't Go Now.   The rejection sensitivity and perceived hostility common to BPD + AUD patients means that patients often have a long list of complaints about AA. Validate their feelings. Focus validation on the emotional impact of prior experiences (e.g., feeling threatened or anxious). Do not challenge the complaints—simply listen, and contain the patient's affect. It will help to "run the well dry" by continuing to ask for more complaints or criticisms. Ideally, the patient will run out of disapprovals. Often, they will then be open to joint consideration of alternative perspectives and interpretations.

Listen for interpersonal hypersensitivity in the patient's narrative. For example, an AA member might offer an AA slogan such as "keep it simple." BPD + AUD patients can take these as criticisms. Think it through with the patient, contextualize it, and tentatively offer interpretations (e.g., "I could be wrong, but perhaps she was trying to connect with you or help you in some way. Is that possible?"). If the patient strongly struggles to consider alternative perspectives, introducing AA reinvolvement is unlikely to work and may harm the therapeutic alliance. Several sessions may be needed to run the well dry. In addition, examine prior involvement much like prior treatments would be assessed:

- What did they not like about AA? What did they like?
- Why did they start or stop going?
- Did they have a sponsor, and how much step work did they complete?
- Did their sponsor read the Big Book with them for step work?
- Did they have any problems with the sponsor?
- What were the relationships like with fellow AA members?
  - Did they participate in fellowship (e.g., coffee/food before or after meetings)
  - Did they have any conflicts?
  - Did they date other AA members?
- Did they attend AA meetings, and if so how many?
- Did they have a home group? What were the demographics?
- How do they feel about the concept of a higher power?

Still Drinking/Relapsing. AA welcomes people struggling to stay sober. Even so, overpowering shame can prevent the patient from continued involvement. This may indicate a need for a higher level of care, but it can also reflect underinvolvement. Examine the patient's reliance on AA to help with cravings. Uncover what prevents them from asking for help from AA members or their sponsor. Identify areas of dishonesty by omission (e.g., hiding cravings). Shame and alexithymia often drive subtle self-deceptions that lead to relapse. Encourage the patient to find another AA member with a history of relapse who is now in successful recovery. Ensure that the patient is sharing at meetings or with AA members about their struggle staying sober.

See later section "Tools for Multimodal Treatment" for a discussion of genograms, home groups, and sponsors.

Skills Training Groups

Skills training groups target self-regulation and interpersonal functioning. The most widely available skills training groups use dialectical behavior therapy (DBT), an evidence-based modality for treating symptoms of BPD (chronic suicidal ideation and behavior). DBT for substance use disorders is an adaptation developed to address co-occurring substance use disorders (Dimeff and Linehan 2008). These groups are run by trained clinicians who provide directive structure and psychoeducation, which may be preferred by some patients. DBT's training-like approach to correct self-regulatory and interpersonal handicaps is compatible with the principles of GPM.

Family Interventions

Family members are an essential part of the social network, and family involvement in the treatment of patients with BPD + AUD can serve a vital function. The symptoms of BPD and AUD impact not only the patient, but also the people in the patient's life. Family and friends may feel helpless and at a loss for how to help their loved one. They may also feel frustrated, angry, or that they are walking on eggshells. They may struggle with how to talk about the patient's alcohol use. It is important to validate the family's difficult experiences living with an individual with BPD + AUD. Families appreciate psychoeducation about the BPD + AUD diagnosis and guidance on how to best support their loved one, which may include advice on parenting skills and recommendations for MHOs, such as Family Connections, Al-Anon, Alateen, SMART Recovery-Family (Table 8–9), or other family-targeted therapeutic approaches, such as Community Reinforcement and Family Training (CRAFT) (Table 8–10). Whereas Al-Anon recommends "loving detachment" from the individual with AUD, CRAFT promotes an approach that is similar to GPM's "leaning in" and providing guidance on effectively engaging (or responding in a different way) with individuals with BPD or AUD. CRAFT is an evidence-based approach for the family members of individuals with AUD (or another substance use disorder) that results in increased rates of patient engagement in AUD treatment and improved quality of life for family members (see Table 8–11) (Meyers et al. 2002; Miller et al. 1999; Roozen et al. 2010).

Enlisting Patient Support for Family Participation

When someone with BPD + AUD initially resists family involvement, they generally are more amenable when it is made clear that the intended

Table 8–9. Mutual-help organizations for families

Diagnosis	Organization	Description
AUD	Al-Anon, Alateen (for teenagers; groups run by Al-Anon adult members who are certified Alateen group sponsors)	12-step program for families (acknowledgment of the powerlessness to change family member with AUD), spiritually based, peer-led
	Families Anonymous	12-step program for families, peer-led
	Adult Children of Alcoholics (ACoA)	12-step program for families, peer-led
BPD	Family Connections	12-class course focused on psychoeducation about BPD, skills training, and support

Note. AUD = alcohol use disorder; BPD = borderline personality disorder.

Table 8–10. Family-targeted intervention

Community Reinforcement and Family Training (CRAFT)	Evidence-based approach for engaging AUD treatment-unengaged individuals by providing support, skills training, and communication training to family members. Promotes self-empowerment of family members. Core features: contingency management, positive reinforcement of healthy or desirable behaviors, avoiding protective behaviors in response to drinking consequences, communication skills training, focus on family members' quality of life.

Note. AUD = alcohol use disorder.
Source. Data from Smith and Myers 2023.

goals are to help their loved ones gain a better understanding of their difficulties and develop a more supportive and less stressful relationship. However, they may continue to resist if they do not see their drinking behavior as problematic or they lack desire to change their problematic BPD-related or drinking behaviors.

Enlisting Family Participation

Clinicians must validate the difficult experiences that family members endure living with an individual with BPD + AUD. Their loved one's symptoms and life may seem unmanageable, and they often feel power-

Table 8–11. GPM guidelines for families

Guideline	Steps	Overlap with CRAFT principles and procedures
Goals: go slowly	1. Change is difficult and fraught with fears 2. Lower expectations; set realistic goals	• Goal setting
Family environment	3. Keep things cool and calm; tone down appreciation and disagreement 4. Maintain family routines; stay in touch with family and friends 5. Find time to talk; chats about light or neutral matters are helpful	• Improving communication skills • Helping family members improve their own lives
Managing crises: pay attention, but stay calm	6. Don't get defensive in the face of accusations or criticisms; say little, don't fight, allow yourself to be hurt 7. Self-destructive acts require attention; don't ignore or panic; talk about it openly 8. Listen; people need to have their negative feelings heard	• Proscriptive behaviors • Avoiding negative reactions • Honest, productive communications
Addressing problems: collaborate and be consistent	9. Three "musts" for solving family problems: a) involve the family member in identifying what needs to be done; b) ask whether the person can do what's needed in the solution; c) ask whether they want you to help them do what's needed 10. Family members: act in concert; parental inconsistencies fuel severe family conflicts 11. Communications with therapist/doctor; if you have concerns about the treatment plan, communicate with family member and treatment team	• Problem-solving • Rewarding non-using behavior • Avoiding protection of drinking consequences

Table 8–11. GPM guidelines for families (*continued*)

Guideline	Steps	Overlap with CRAFT principles and procedures
Limit setting: be direct but careful	12. Set limits, limits of your tolerance. Set clear expectations in simple language. 13. Don't protect from natural consequences—allow them to learn about reality. Bumping into a few walls is usually necessary. 14. Don't tolerate abusive treatment—walk away and return to discuss the issue later. 15. Be cautious about using threats and ultimatums. They are a last resort.	• Allowing for the natural, negative consequences of use • Avoiding threatening and other punitive responses to drinking-related problems

Note. CRAFT = Community Reinforcement and Family Training; GPM = good psychiatric management.
Source. Data from Gunderson and Berkowitz 2006; Smith and Myers 2023.

less to help, which is potentially how the patient feels as well (i.e., parallel process). Family members are aware that what they have been doing has not worked, and they may be willing to try something new.

Alliance Building

The symptoms of BPD + AUD worsen family dysfunction and vice versa. Hence, intervening at the level of the family may help ameliorate the symptoms of both BPD and AUD. To start, GPM and CRAFT both recommend building alliances through offering support, psychoeducation including skill building, and collaboration.

Support for Family Members

Family members of those with BPD + AUD may feel alone as they deal with emotional distress and financial burden. It is important to listen and validate their difficult experiences, which may include fears of suicide, destruction of the family unit, and legal or medical consequences of their loved one's BPD-related behaviors and alcohol use. While reassuring them that they have tried their best, let them know that the patient's deficits stemming from BPD and AUD require a different response.

Psychoeducation

Psychoeducation is a core principle of GPM that is continually emphasized throughout the treatment with the patient and the family. Once they have a better understanding of the disorders, family members can begin to make sense of the symptoms of BPD and AUD, which are often initially confusing, and be in a better position to respond in a way that helps (see Table 8–12 for communication guidelines). Next, we provide a sample dialogue explaining the complex interaction between genetic and environmental factors contributing to the development of these disorders, as well as the neurobiological overlap between them. This information provides a medical framework and moves away from assigning blame, which is often associated with shame.

> The development of both BPD and AUD stems from an interaction between genetics and environment. Both are significantly heritable psychiatric conditions. Individuals with strong genetic predispositions are more vulnerable to developing these disorders when faced with environmental adversity. Although the details are not fully understood, the BPD patient likely inherited either excessive emotionality or interpersonal reactivity that leads to a difficult temperament to parent. Hence, BPD gen-

Table 8–12. Positive communication guidelines

1. Be brief.
2. Use positive/action-oriented wording.
3. Mention specific behaviors.
4. Label your feelings.
5. Offer an understanding statement.
6. Accept partial responsibility (for something related to the situation, not for the substance use).
7. Offer to help.

Source.   Smith JE, Myers RJ: The CRAFT Treatment Manual for Substance Use Problems: Working With Family Members. New York, Guilford Press, 2023. Reprinted with permission of Guilford Press.

erally develops when there is a mismatch between temperamental needs of the patient and parental responses. In both BPD and AUD, there is likely an inherited stress vulnerability.

Individuals with BPD often lack appropriate coping skills and may engage in impulsive and self-destructive acts, such as drinking alcohol or self-injury, to self-regulate or communicate distress. Alcohol use can worsen BPD symptoms and vice versa—BPD and AUD include overlapping neurobiological dysfunctions, including an overactive limbic system, underactive prefrontal cortex, and dysregulation ("hijacking") of the brain's reward/pleasure centers.

Many families may ask about the role of trauma and development of these disorders:

A significant number of individuals with BPD and a substance use disorder such as AUD report a childhood adverse event or history of trauma. It is thought that such events contribute to the etiology but are neither necessary nor sufficient for development of these disorders.

Families also ask about the prognosis of each disorder and how they can help:

BPD+AUD patients do improve with treatment. You can help promote the recovery of your loved one by providing support that is in line with the GPM guidelines for families (see Table 8–11).

Collaboration and Skills Building

An essential part of the social network for a patient with BPD+AUD is collaboration among the family, patient, and treatment team. Psychoeducation should take place first. Then, with an understanding of the BPD+AUD patient's interpersonal hypersensitivity, limited self-control, and pattern of alcohol use, the family should provide basic support that is consistent with GPM guidelines (Table 8–13). The family must understand that change is slow and that goals for treatment must be realistic. Patients with BPD+AUD may exhibit anger toward family members as well as criticize and blame them, but it is important not to take it too personally or fight back. In these cases, tolerate the symptoms to a degree, but set limits and allow for natural consequences. Family members must prioritize their safety and well-being. Living or caring for someone with BPD+AUD is challenging. Family members should strive to be "good enough" supports.

Family members can tailor how they respond to and engage with BPD+AUD patients with the help of the family guidelines (Table 8–11) as well as positive communication guidelines (Table 8–12). Considering the disruptive and self-destructive behaviors of patients with BPD+AUD, they often do not hear anything positive. An effort by family members to modify how they communicate with BPD+AUD individuals may have an impact. In addition, rewarding healthy behaviors, such as not drinking, can serve as positive reinforcement that can shape behavior over time and serve to promote recovery.

Common Problems in Family Intervention

Your Patient Refuses to Allow Contact With Family Members

Family members are an important part of the social network for the patient with BPD+AUD. Family members can provide helpful information pertaining to concerns and tracking of progress. Although confidentiality of the BPD+AUD patient must be respected, treaters must communicate that family involvement and support are typically necessary for successful treatment.

The Family Does Not Adhere to Family Guidelines

Family members may relapse to old habits. Return to motivational interviewing about the pros and cons of trying to foster the patient's recovery despite setbacks or discouragements, with the goal of family members recommitting to the guidelines. Change is difficult to achieve, and the process is fraught with fears. Clinicians may need to lower expectations,

Table 8–13. Hierarchy of family interventions for patients with BPD + AUD[a]

Type of intervention	Features	Comments
Psychoeducation	Focus on understanding BPD + AUD and the prognosis	For family guidelines, see Table 8–11
Counseling/family-targeted interventions	Review family guidelines; advise; problem-solve; see Table 8–10 (CRAFT)	Families usually welcome these sessions
Mutual-help groups	Multiple family groups, Al-Anon, Alateen, Families Anonymous, Family Connections[b]	Helpful if available; see Table 8–9 for description of each group
Conjoint sessions (patients and family/friends)	Useful for planning and problem-solving issues such as budget, sleep hygiene, treatment adherence, emergencies, vacations	Can be very helpful in sustaining the holding environment and to decrease splitting
Family therapy	Reserved for patients and parents; discuss conflicts without interrupting, having angry outbursts, or leaving	Confronting parental caretaking failures may be useful only if parents can accept with regret mistakes of the past without losing hope for future improvement

Note. AUD = alcohol use disorder; BPD = borderline personality disorder; CRAFT = Community Reinforcement and Family Training.
[a]In terms of availability, breadth of identity, and costs.
[b]Family Connections is sponsored by National Education Alliance for Borderline Personality Disorder/National Alliance on Mental Illness.
Source. Adapted from Gunderson and Links 2014.

set realistic goals, and solve problems in small steps. Overly large, long-term goals can lead to discouragement and failure.

Tools for Multimodal Treatment

Genogram: Family History of Alcohol Use

The genogram is an illustration that medicalizes alcohol abuse as a disease that can be traced across generations, rather than a moral failure or character flaw. It has the benefits of contextualizing the patient's alcohol use, connecting it to subjective experiences, and providing valuable information to the clinician that can be accessed in future therapeutic work. A whiteboard or large piece of paper is used to collaboratively contemplate the drinking behavior and consequences of the patient and family members across three generations (i.e., the patient's parents, the patient and siblings, and children). Essentially, the genogram is designed to open a conversation about how alcohol abuse has harmed the patient, other family members, and the patient's relationships. For example, this could include instances where the patient felt shame about a parent's drinking (*my mom picked me up at school and my friends teased me that she smelled like alcohol*), consequences of the patient's drinking (*I am broke, in liver failure, and homeless*), and impact on the patient's relationships (*my wife left me, saying she could not watch me drink myself to death*).

Importantly, the hypersensitivity inherent in patients with BPD + AUD can lead to overwhelming emotions during the process of constructing the genogram. Be watchful of subtle shifts in body posture, eye contact, and intonation. These might be clues that the patient is becoming too activated and needs a break. The discomfort in confronting the family history of alcohol use can lead the patient away from discussing specific situations, behaviors, and consequences related to drinking. Avoidance can surface as detailed storytelling and topic shifting. Taking a break and steering the patient back toward a structured discussion of alcohol use will create a holding environment and keep the discussion focused on the impact of alcohol within the family.

After completing the genogram, session time should be dedicated to discussing the patient's general experience of the genogram. (*What was it like to think about this? How did you feel while talking through the family's history of drinking?*) Throughout the session, BPD + AUD patients may experience dissociative symptoms presenting as dismissiveness of the genogram and family history. Later that day, they can be vulnerable to overwhelming emotions. The clinician and patient can prospectively cope through this phenomenon by jointly considering how the genogram might impact the patient later. Discuss strategies the patient can use to soothe themselves after the session, such as increasing social support.

The Therapeutic Environment of Home Groups

A home group is an AA meeting, or AA meeting location (e.g., church, AA club), where the patient is accountable, learns about AA, finds a sponsor, develops skills to rely on the AA fellowship, and can begin experiencing stable relationships. As the patient starts attending a home group consistently, the members come to expect the patient's presence. Frequently, members communicate this expectation of attendance (*I didn't see you last week, how are you?*). Although a question like this can trigger an experience of shame, it is often asked thoughtfully, and BPD + AUD patients experience a sense of containment and connectedness. It expresses to the patient that they were remembered, considered, and wanted. Over time, patients will believe that AA home group members are authentically interested in them and their experience. This opens a learning channel between AA members and the patient.

The transfer of wisdom between AA home group members mirrors many of GPM's principles and interventions. For example, the patient might say to a home group member, *I spent all day in my head, worrying about my boyfriend.* Home group members often respond therapeutically: *I can totally relate* (validation). *Did you call anyone in the program?* (accountability). *That always helps me* (expectation of change).

This straightforward response validates the unbearable mental state of the BPD + AUD patient as understandable, common, and fixable. Simultaneously, it holds the frame of AA (i.e., that the patient is accountable to addressing the problem—in this case, apparent rumination) and an expectation of change (i.e., in the future, calling an AA member can help). This increases the patient's hope and commitment to the AA program. They have expressed themselves honestly, openly, and willingly. Someone they trust has responded sensitively with a practical solution. This example illustrates the impact of having a home group with an active learning environment.

While listening to several (or several dozen) members share during the meeting, the BPD + AUD patient hears how members actively navigate cognitive challenges (e.g., black-and-white thinking), affective states (e.g., painful emotions), and behavioral precursors to alcohol use (e.g., dishonesty). The patient learns that members address these vulnerabilities through increased social support. A member might share how she called her sponsor when feeling anxious or threatened—her sponsor listened to her, validated her experience, and suggested practical solutions. Most meetings follow the format of sharing personal experience. Comments or advice toward specific members is prohibited and reserved for pre/post-meeting fellowship. This format provides a safe environment for BPD+AUD patients that allows increasingly transparent honesty in the context of overpowering shame.

Broadly, AA members refer to AA meetings as either problem-based or solution-based meetings. Problem-based meetings focus on detailed histories of drinking with little reference to sponsorship, the 12 steps, or behavioral change. Solution-based meetings place heavy emphasis on sponsorship, working and completing the 12 steps with a sponsor, practical solutions to everyday problems, and life in recovery. Encourage patients to find solution-based meetings.

In solution-based meetings, home group members contact their sponsors regularly and share about working the steps as outlined in the AA basic text (the Big Book). There will be years of sobriety among home group members. Members will approach the patient when they first attend, welcome them warmly, and engage them in conversation. These welcoming behaviors show that the meeting is empathic and outwardly focused on the new members. Alongside welcoming the newcomer, solution-based meetings have service jobs available such as pouring coffee, setting up/cleaning up, or being meeting secretary, front door greeter, literature representative, sponsorship representative, treasurer, and service coordinator. Service coordinators serve as liaisons between the home group and service commitments such as speaking at hospitals, penitentiaries, and other meetings. Through sharing at these service commitments, the patient learns how to provide psychoeducation about AA/alcoholism and is an active and accountable participant in the recovery process. Moreover, BPD+AUD patients can have their first salutogenic experiences, such as increases in self-esteem through the act of helping others. Assess the quality of the meeting by asking specific questions about these features, leading with curiosity and humility.

> I've read a little about AA meetings and what makes an AA meeting good. I was hoping you could tell me more? What was it like to attend this meeting? What were the people like? Could you identify with what they shared? Were there sponsors available? Does the meeting have service commitments?

The Sponsor As a Second Treater

When overlaid on GPM, good sponsorship mirrors GPM's three forms of therapeutic alliance: contractual, relational, and working alliance.

Contractually, the first conversations with a potential sponsor outline the AA framework. For example, the sponsor might say:

> I would be happy to work with you. My job is to complete the 12 steps with you as outlined in the Big Book. I expect you call me rather than text me, and to meet with me once a week to read and write out of the Big Book. When we're finished with the 12 steps, I expect you to bring another alcoholic through the 12 steps.

This highlights the goals of AA and helps the BPD + AUD patient feel psychologically contained through knowing what to expect, their own role, and the role of their sponsor. Sponsors can vary in initial expectations (e.g., frequency of phone calls), but every effective sponsor will center the relationship around working the 12 steps. As with GPM, when the contractual alliance fails, another sponsor might be more helpful.

Relationally, sponsors often lead with empathic validation. Initial conversations focus on identification of shared experiences, expressions of understanding, and instillation of hope. For example:

> I get it, and I have been there. When I joined AA, my husband would not speak to me or let me see the kids. It was terrible. I just kept coming back to AA because I did not know what to do. When I got a sponsor and started working the steps, I started to understand why I drank, and today I have the closest relationship with my kids that I've ever had.

Given a shared background and identification with consequences of alcohol use, the sponsor is uniquely positioned to convey authentic warmth and hope. This lays the foundation for change-oriented work in the steps.

The working alliance focuses on step work. After meeting the contractual expectations and coming to believe the sponsor has shared experience, the sponsee is far more likely to take direction. The alliance is characterized by weekly meetings with a focus on step work, but it also provides acute problem-solving and the opportunity for necessary feedback. For example,

> You have been talking a lot about what he said and did. Isn't it true that you called him names before all this?

While this kind of comment may seem risky, AA sponsors are often allowed the most latitude with BPD + AUD patients. Over time, patients begin to simulate "what their sponsor might say," and this can be leveraged within psychotherapeutic work.

Conclusion

Multimodal treatments expand and enhance the social networks of BPD + AUD patients with psychotherapy groups (e.g., DBT, mentalization-based therapy, schema-focused therapy), MHOs (e.g., AA, Smart Recovery, LifeRing), and active family involvement.

Social networks capitalize on the basic human need to form and maintain close relationships, creating a protective net against symptomatic and functional declines. Through an in vivo process of social learning, BPD + AUD patients obtain immediate support, identify with their peers, develop problem-solving skills, learn to manage vulnerabilities, build identities, and have corrective experiences. Psychotherapy groups are a safe environment that instill hope of recovery while reducing shame and increasing self-understanding. Active AA involvement increases the probability of long-term abstinence and full remission of AUD while supporting active efforts at personality change. The GPM-AUD clinician can guide family relationships toward approaches that promote recovery while addressing corrosive family dynamics. Altogether, facilitating these changes in the social network of the BPD + AUD patient provides a foundation for recovery while scaffolding and supporting the treater, thereby increasing the chances of treatment success and reducing the likelihood of clinician burnout and failed treatments.

9

Level-of-Care Considerations for Patients With Substance Use Disorder and Borderline Personality Disorder

Robin Gay, Ph.D.
Hilary S. Connery, M.D., Ph.D.

This chapter is intended to guide clinicians in selecting appropriate levels of care for patients with co-occurring borderline personality disorder (BPD) and alcohol use disorder (AUD). The American Society for Addiction Medicine Criteria (ASAM Criteria) derive from an evidence-based algorithm developed to standardize and capture levels of functioning and care needs among patients with substance use disorders (SUDs) and currently serves as the gold standard for determining SUD patient level-of-care (LOC) placement. In brief, the ASAM Criteria have five main levels of care (0–4) and uses a dimensional model to score symptom severity within each LOC.

ASAM was founded in 1954, and the original criteria were published in 1991 to provide consistent decision-making concerning the treatment needs that would be effective and least restrictive for SUD patients. Since then, the algorithm has been developed further to capture complex social, medical, and co-occurring mental health needs of SUD patients. Although mental health considerations are part of the algorithm, the criteria do not specifically consider the unique care needs of patients with both BPD and SUDs.

There is no evidence-based equivalent algorithm for LOC placement for BPD. As such, we interpret the structural benefits of the ASAM Criteria that may be applied within a good psychiatric management (GPM) model of care for BPD with co-occurring AUD (GPM-AUD), while acknowledging that LOC decision-making for BPD+AUD may have competing factors (e.g., the need to admit a patient for withdrawal management of AUD competing with the goal of keeping BPD patients functioning independently in outpatient care). The ASAM Criteria are well suited for adaptation to patients with BPD, as both BPD and AUD disorders occur on a spectrum of functionality. SUDs have dimensional specifiers (mild to severe, depending on number of AUD symptom criteria met during the past year; see Chapter 4, "Making the Diagnosis"), with minimal impairment in functioning to more severe functional impairment (e.g., job loss, alienation from family, and health consequences including premature death due to organ failure, injury, unintentional poisoning, and suicide). BPD symptom severity and functional impairment are likewise dimensional, with many patients stable and productive, and some having severe levels of disruption in daily living (occupational and relational), deficits in self-regulation and identity, elevated self-harm behaviors and suicide risk, and time spent in psychiatric hospital settings. Both disorders may have a remitting-relapsing course. Thus, longitudinal treatment must be flexible and responsive to increasing or reducing treatment intensity while maintaining the least restrictive treatment setting that provides safety and preserves autonomy.

Why Adaptation of American Society of Addiction Medicine Levels of Care Helps Guide Standard-of-Care Interventions

Heightened Risk and Maintenance Care Models for Patients With BPD+SUD

Given the paucity of research on treatment and outcomes specific to BPD+AUD patients, and given the challenges of overlapping behavioral and cognitive symptoms in both BPD and AUD presentations, the application of evidence-based standards of care for each disorder provides the best practice model currently available. Available evidence suggests an additive symptom severity and risk profile for patients with BPD+AUD, compared with BPD or AUD alone. These observations may be explained in part by developmental processes that increase stress sensitivity and reduce self-reflective functioning, with consequent maladaptive coping mechanisms that worsen stress sensitivity and capacity for self-reflective functioning. For example, BPD patients with deficits in emotion regulation may use substances in response to emotional reactivity and difficulty managing interpersonal conflict. Generally, substance use further destabilizes the core BPD symptom expression and interferes with psychosocial treatment adherence. Alcohol and other substance use, especially during teenage development, interrupts and impairs consolidation of key developmental skills, such as the ability to self-regulate and tolerate difficult emotions, effectively communicate in high-conflict situations, and maintain daily structure and social connectedness. This diminishes normal identity integration during development and adds risk factors for both unintentional and intentional self-harm behaviors.

Current evidence favors integrated treatment of BPD+AUD for best outcomes. A maintenance care model applies to both BPD and AUD independently and appears to benefit the care of BPD+AUD. For example, Laporte et al. (2018) reported that stepped care interventions matching treatment intensity to symptom severity are effective for BPD, with higher-intensity extended care favoring BPD with significant alcohol misuse as measured by the Addiction Severity Index.

High Community Prevalence of Co-occurring SUDs and BPD

BPD is prevalent in patients with SUDs. Data show that ~14% of current patients diagnosed with BPD have SUDs, and up to 72% of patients diagnosed with BPD have SUDs in their lifetimes. Interestingly, some studies show that among those with SUDs, there are more men than women in treatment with co-occurring BPD; an exception is prescription drug misuse, where rates of men and women with co-occurring BPD are similar. These differences may be an artifact related to women avoiding treatment until SUDs are more severe, due to stigma and parenting concerns. Some studies looking at rates in community samples rather than treatment settings show comparable SUD rates among men and women with BPD.

Importance of the Treatment Level Matching the Level of Clinical Need

Carefully matching the level of treatment with clinical presentation and symptom severity is important for maintenance of functioning, continued progress, and substance use reduction. Sonley and Choi-Kain (2021) introduced a framework for stepped care based on the Chanen et al. (2016) model for patients with BPD. The framework begins with psycho-education, then supportive counseling at preclinical stages; GPM principles, higher levels of care, and traditional treatments are applied to those who do not respond. The model presented here incorporates aspects of this stepped care structure.

Additional areas are considered, including transitions between levels, as progress and patient functioning within each LOC need to be continually assessed. Ascertaining progress, patient adherence, and ability to utilize skills taught to maintain care goals, including substance use reduction and suicide prevention, is a longitudinal and collaborative process. Special care is given to transitions between levels of care, especially from emergency department or acute inpatient and residential settings to ambulatory care, given the increased risk of suicide and substance relapse during these transitions.

Similarities Between Level-of-Care Determinations for SUDs and BPD

Both Are Supportive and Pragmatic

Treatment of SUDs and BPD shares many of the same principles—for example, GPM focuses on "awareness, acceptance, identification of feeling states," which is a skill set that is also emphasized in SUD treatment. GPM is a supportive and pragmatic treatment, as are evidence-based approaches to SUD care (see also Chapter 2, "Overall Principles," and Chapter 3, "Integrating DDP Into GPM"). Initial treatment goals avoid exploratory therapy and prioritize behavioral stabilization with education and cognitive skills training to manage symptoms effectively and reduce self-harm and risk behaviors. Both emphasize engagement with a stable and supportive community as an essential component of good outcome and improved social functioning. Both emphasize autonomy and accountability to goal-setting and behavioral change. Additionally, both emphasize a recovery network that assists social functioning by facilitating vocational structure, stabilizing identity by finding personal meaning as well as social purpose, and living fully according to one's values in the context of positive social connectedness. In this way, both also foster interpersonal talents, needs, interests, and abilities.

American Society for Addiction Medicine Criteria for Substance Use Disorder Patient Placement

ASAM levels of care are shown in Figure 9–1. Within each of these levels, patients are considered on six dimensions and given severity rankings from 0 (no issue) to 4 (highest risk/imminent danger) (Figure 9–2).

Clinicians can assess care needs at each level and adapt these levels to best fit the profile of patients with both SUDs and BPD. Determining and labeling the level of care individuals need provides for consistency of treatment across institutions and different programs. Consistency is an important therapeutic intervention to reduce stress sensitivity and increase treatment engagement for BPD, AUD, and BPD+AUD. Guidance for LOC alleviates anxiety and disputes among providers and payers, and thus reduces burnout for clinicians while achieving swift and appropriate clinical interventions.

General Principles in Determining Levels of Care

Stabilization of safety and functioning, especially when a patient is in crisis or actively misusing substances, is the priority consideration in determining LOC. Other considerations for BPD+AUD include how to determine LOC when symptom severity is stable in one disorder and unstable in the other. In general, if one disorder is substantially more unstable and the focus of risk mitigation, then that should be outlined explicitly in patient care treatment planning, recognizing the dynamic nature of symptom recurrence for both BPD and AUD and tending to prevention of symptom recurrence in the more stable disorder. Placement at a higher LOC for severe BPD (life-threatening symptoms) would be a psychiatric treatment setting, whereas the need for AUD withdrawal management without severe BPD symptom expression may favor a substance use treatment setting. We recommend the use of substance relapse planning in treatment (Figure 9–1), analogous to the evidence-based use of the Stanley-Brown Safety Plan for suicide prevention (Stanley and Brown 2012; https://suicidesafetyplan.com/).

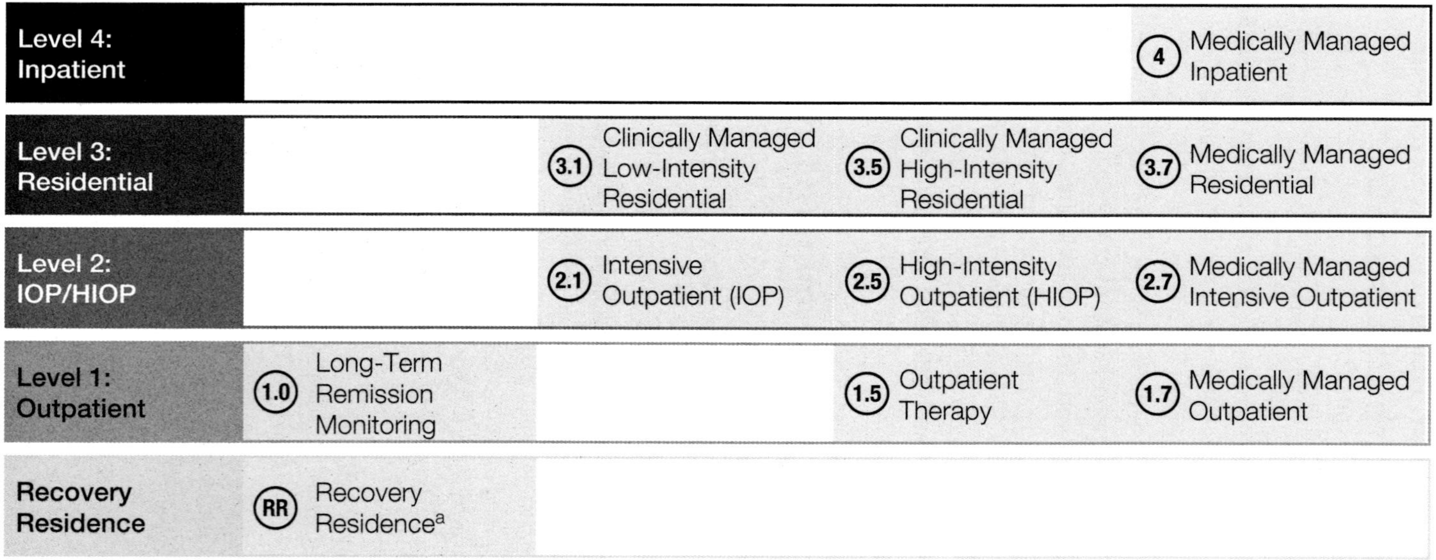

Figure 9–1. *The ASAM Criteria* continuum of care for adult addiction treatment.

[a]Recovery residence may be recommended to provide safe and stable housing to support engagement in outpatient services (Level 1 or 2).
Source. The ASAM Criteria: Treatment for Addictive, Substance-related, and Co-occurring Conditions, 4th Edition. ISBN 979-8-9876803-0-8, copyright 2023, American Society for Addiction Medicine. Reprinted with permission from ASAM.

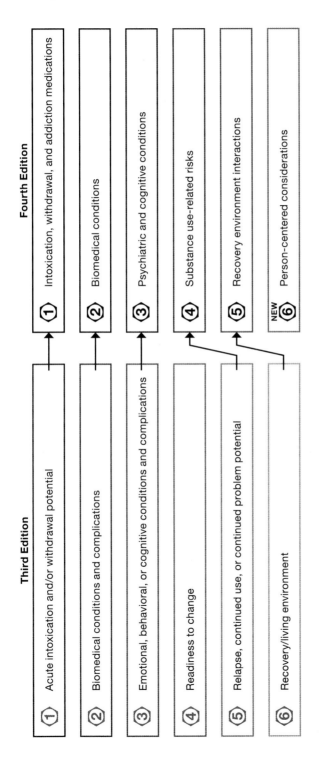

Figure 9-2. Changes to the ASAM Criteria with the 4th Edition

Source. The ASAM Criteria: Treatment for Addictive, Substance-related, and Co-occurring Conditions, 4th Edition. ISBN 979-8-9876803-0-8, copyright 2023, American Society for Addiction Medicine. Reprinted with permission from ASAM.

Using a Higher Level of Care Than Needed Can Impede Progress

Levels of care need to be fluid to adapt to the patient's current needs; they also should be the least restrictive possible for a given phase of care, to allow for the greatest level of autonomous, independent functioning. Using higher levels of care to manage a patient's intolerance of aloneness and impulsive states can delay their success in self-reliance and community connection. Overused higher levels of care have been shown to have negative outcomes for long-term independent functioning in patients with BPD (Gunderson and Links 2008; Knight 1953; Quaytman and Sharfstein 1997). Similarly, ASAM studies for SUDs indicated that briefer-duration intensive treatments are not inferior to longer-duration residential care (although extended residential care may be appropriate for those who do not sustain gains from briefer treatments). For BPD + AUD, there is convergent best practice to institute higher LOC for acute safety stabilization and then step treatment down as stabilization is achieved.

Continuum of Care Rather Than Discrete Episodes

Treatment models for SUDs focus on a continuum of care rather than discrete treatment episodes. TIP 47 from the Substance Abuse and Mental Health Services Administration advocates that programs adopt a language for continuum of care and that programs "envision admitting the client into the continuum through their program rather than admitting the client to their program" (SAMHSA 2006). TIPS explains that this language helps patients prepare for the possibility of ongoing levels of care throughout their lives. The language aids patients who have both BPD and SUDs, as it conceives of treatment as an ongoing process in which transient changes to the intensity of care are required for good outcome. Conceptualizing treatment on a continuum is also beneficial for patients and families, as there may be a misconception that treatment will last for a specific duration (for example, 30 days, in the case of residential treatment), with a misunderstanding that completion of this treatment episode will cure the illness.

Discussing levels of care early in treatment is beneficial psychoeducation. Offering clear guidance and expectations facilitates predictability and collaborative decision-making between the patient, family, and treatment team. In outlining symptom severity and safety thresholds that trigger consideration of LOC changes, such discussion also reduces disputes among care team providers regarding changes to treatment intensity.

Institutional preferences of BPD+AUD patients are important to consider in treatment planning (Figure 9–1), while acknowledging that admissions availability is not predictable; thus a ranked list of treatment options may be needed. Making such a list also has the advantage of anticipating patient or family devaluation of one treatment center over another and resolving an algorithmic approach to disposition that includes patient and family preferences during crisis interventions. Patients and families are educated to expect that, for smooth transitions and optimal outcomes, referring clinicians need to share information with those who are providing higher-intensity services.

It is important that all care team providers are aware of the LOC framework and agree on how LOC transitions will be executed. Any potential disagreements are best resolved before meeting with the patient. For example, a therapy patient with attachment trauma and poor emotional regulation may become more symptomatic if a withdrawal management admission is required for safe stabilization. In this case, a psychiatric treatment setting would be favored over a substance use disorder treatment setting. To promote agency and be consistent with a containing environment, try to anticipate possible future scenarios and develop a plan in advance with the patient.

Reassessing Patients With Substance Use Disorders and Borderline Personality Disorder: Step-Ups and Step-Downs in Care

Patients with both SUDs and BPD may have sudden changes in functioning. It is important to proactively assess for warning signs and triggers, as patients can sometimes deteriorate rapidly. The goal is for the patient to be able to identify warning signs and effectively use skills to manage self-harm and substance use recurrence. During acute deterioration, any point of care may be an entry into treatment for timely risk mitigation. For example, patients functioning well in ambulatory care may experience rapid deterioration because of unexpected life circumstances or a loss, and in such circumstances the patient may be seen urgently in an ambulatory setting or may present to an emergency department for evaluation. The aim is for a nimble response within the care continuum to quickly contain safety risks.

It is important for clinicians and patients alike not to pathologize these transitions or conceptualize them as failures. Often patients become focused on perceived failures when they need to re-enter a higher LOC, and this can be a major impediment for treatment. Clinicians can help patients view these LOC adjustments as an expected part of the recovery process. Here again, the continuum model of stepped levels of care can help alleviate the perceived stigma of needing to re-enter a higher LOC, reframing the transition as evidence that the patient is committed to recovery and self-care.

ASAM Patient Placement Criteria Applications for BPD + AUD

Early Intervention, ASAM Level 0.5

Early intervention is arguably the most important LOC, as it has the possibility of intervening before a full disorder develops. The lifetime prevalence for any individual being diagnosed with AUD is surprisingly high, at 29.1% (Grant et al. 2015); according to the 2021 National Survey on Drug Use and Health study, 10.6% of all individuals 12 or older met criteria for AUD. Patients with BPD make up a substantial proportion of those with SUDs who seek treatment. Among patients with AUD, the most prevalent co-occurring conditions are depression, bipolar disorder, antisocial personality disorder, and BPD.

Screening

ASAM criteria at this level focus on screening patients and identifying those who may benefit from preventive interventions. Screening for substance misuse is easily integrated into routine BPD care, giving clinicians the opportunity to address risky use and prevent it from progressing to an SUD. Routine screening can help identify those at risk, as well as those who already have a problem but have not sought treatment. Psychoeducation and screening at this stage are helpful—many do not seek treatment until the disorder is severe, with negative social and health consequences. Evidence-based screens include the three-item Alcohol Use Disorders Identification Test-Concise (AUDIT-C) for problematic alcohol use (see Appendix E; see also Chapter 4, "Making the Diagnosis"). The McLean Screening Instrument for Borderline Personality Disorder is a 10-item brief screen that may be considered for screening the general population (Zanarini et al. 2003). Early intervention decreases mortality and course severity for both BPD and SUDs.

Psychoeducation: Individual and Family

After identifying someone at risk, the first intervention is to provide normative feedback and psychoeducation that engages a patient in care. For some, this may be enough to stop risky drinking from progressing to AUD. Likewise, for some patients with BPD, early psychoeducation provided to the family can be extremely beneficial. For example, a family can learn ways to better validate their child's or teen's emotional experience by taking a nonjudgmental stance, without pathologizing their emotions, and at the same time not reinforcing maladaptive behaviors. Education is important for the family, providing tools for coping with stress without using substances. Psychoeducation for families regarding treatment for substance misuse and SUD is also beneficial (see Appendices C and D).

Level 1, Outpatient Treatment

Outpatient care has the widest number of options, with many types of support. This level of care is important in that it fosters autonomy and self-direction. The patient is expected to actively assess what types of outpatient treatment they believe will be most helpful. Outpatient care commonly consists of individual psychotherapy and psychopharmacology; it may also include recovery coaching, community supports, recovery groups, monitoring devices (breathalyzer or toxicology screening), and digital treatment supports. This level of care is best suited for patients who can self-regulate, identify triggers, and know how and when to reach out for extra support when necessary. Patients need to utilize skills to avoid relapse and regulate emotions. Patients are trained to anticipate situations that may be challenging and to develop strategies and plans to manage and cope with those stressors. Outpatient care is inadequate for patients with frequent and severe self-harm behaviors or life-threatening substance use.

Outpatient Group Treatment

Patients with BPD + AUD often benefit from participation in group therapies. There are many groups available for patients with BPD or SUDs, and some groups specifically for both. Some benefits of group treatment include the connection with others that is inherent in a group setting, learning healthy communication techniques, having the opportunity to practice and receive peer feedback, and receiving support from others who have similar experiences. Patients may experience interpersonal hypersensitivity that can best be processed in a group format, as patients can use group dynamics to achieve better reality testing. Patients can test out their hypothesis with other group members and obtain valuable feedback. Groups are also beneficial as they may offer an experience of re-parenting and good-enough holding. Good-enough consistency of expectations of self and others may also be achieved, as groups help foster development and practice of needed social skills and self-acceptance. Group treatment is inherently skill building and helps with self-awareness (see also Chapter 8, "Multimodal Treatments").

Other Options: Sober Coaching, Apps, and Substance Monitoring

Although the concept of having a sponsor has been around for quite some time, sober coaching in the United States began on the West Coast about 20 years ago. Sober coaching is a valuable type of treatment that focuses on accountability and skills building with an interpersonal viewpoint. Coaches, who are in sustained substance recovery themselves, have received training and achieved certification. The difference from a 12-step sponsor is that the coach's goal is to meet the individual where they are and adjust their services to the individual's preferences. An additional benefit is that they are generally available 24 hours a day if needed and are able to offer brief daily contacts. As such, the approach is hands-on and tailored to the client's needs.

There are now multiple digital applications (apps) to help manage symptoms of SUDs and BPD (see Appendix D). Patients must engage with these programs regularly for them to be effective. Devices (such as breathalyzers) can measure point-of-care urine or saliva toxicology in real time. These tools can assist patients who are engaged in care but still need external accountability supports. Such monitoring needs to be structured to support care and should not be used to "catch" patients or justify care withdrawal.

Sober Homes/Supportive Living

Sober homes/group homes are often adjuncts to outpatient treatment. Patients in sober homes or group homes participate in individual psychotherapy and psychopharmacology, as well as more intensive ambulatory treatment programs. Individuals who come to treatment from an environment that is risky or triggering (such as drugs or alcohol being used by others in the home) may not be able to go home because of the risk of relapse or difficulty regulating emotions and behaviors. A sober home, besides being an environment without substances, helps a patient to exit a family or home environment that may be contributing to illness severity. A sober home allows time for family dynamics to change and communication skills to improve before the patient returns. Additionally, sober/group homes work well for individuals who were not functioning well living alone. These types of homes create and provide a holding environment and reinforce prosocial, goal-oriented behaviors, which can be especially helpful for those at risk of using or experiencing dysregulated emotional states. These facilities provide structure and an environment where patients can live with others who have common goals.

Expectations in these homes are clear and consistent, and if boundaries are crossed or rules violated, there are clearly defined consequences. In this way, patients are motivated, in a positive manner, to achieve and conform to community standards for social accountability. Some residential or sober homes have a system in which patients enter an intensively structured home with heavy oversight, and as they improve in that environment they may step down or "graduate" to a home with far less oversight and structure. These LOC transitions consider how well an individual can tolerate discomfort (related to both substance cravings and emotional distress) in a structured yet highly independent environment. The individual should be able to identify their own emotional states, be aware of potential high-risk situations, and be ready to ask for help when needed.

Level 2, Intensive Outpatient/Partial Hospitalization

For patients who need more intensive ambulatory treatment services—particularly for those who have just ended residential care or inpatient hospitalization—intensive outpatient programs (IOPs) and partial hospital programs (PHPs, also referred to as day treatment) may be useful. Patients returning to their home environment need a gradual easing (titrating) of services. This level of care provides multiple group sessions per week alongside individual treatment planning. This level is best for individuals who are still learning to manage dysregulated affect, conflictual relationship patterns, or substance cravings and who are actively engaged in developing and practicing new skills. The benefit is that they can learn these skills and have daily or weekly contact with their treatment team should any problems arise.

Level 3, Residential/Inpatient

This level of care is best suited for patients who need additional support, who need a monitored environment that restricts access to substances and dangerous people, and who can benefit from the highly structured treatments provided. After the emotional experience of BPD or long-term use of substances, patients may have a poorly defined sense of self, and their mood may be labile owing to paranoid projections and rejection hypersensitivity. The consistent and supportive environment provided by residential and inpatient care addresses impaired social relating as well as development of more effective substance relapse prevention skills. This context offers environmental protection and safety in which to re-evaluate treatment goals and self-care skills with the help of clinicians and peers.

Level 4, Medically Managed Intensive Inpatient

According to ASAM criteria, Level 4 is for patients who need withdrawal management from substances and require 24-hour medical treatment. For BPD, this level of care equivalent would be for patients who are in imminent danger of acute self-harm or suicidal behavior. In both cases, units may be locked for safe containment while the patient is medically and behaviorally stabilized, with discharge to a lower LOC once stable. Duration of care is intentionally brief, often less than 1 week.

Conclusion

Throughout each of the levels of care, the frame and structure help model development of internal structure that is an important goal of treatment for patients with BPD+AUD. Effective care management involves contingency planning that anticipates fluctuating phases of symptom severity and health risks. The use of clearly outlined patient and family care coordination and treatment agreements may assist in communication, collaborative decision-making in stepped care, and provider agreement across LOC transitions.

10

Putting It Together in the Real World: Tips for Adapting GPM-AUD to Your Clinical Setting

Hilary S. Connery, M.D., Ph.D.
Lois W. Choi-Kain, M.D., M.Ed.

We wrote this final chapter to give behavioral health care clinicians and nonspecialist providers some tips on practical implementation of good psychiatric management of borderline personality disorder and alcohol use disorder (GPM-AUD). Here we address common reasons that clinicians avoid treatment of both borderline personality disorder (BPD) and substance use disorder (SUD) populations, and we offer realistic "good-enough" solutions to providing care confidently. We also briefly discuss the treatment of patients with BPD and co-occurring SUDs. Risk mitigation is emphasized throughout.

Clinician Avoidance Derives From Liability Fears and Feeling Personally Manipulated

Many studies have examined stigma, bias, and barriers to care for BPD and SUDs (for example, see Klein et al. 2022 [BPD] and Kelly et al. 2021 [SUDs]). Common stigmatizing attitudes of clinicians toward BPD patients reflect aversion to recurrent crisis presentations, high suicide risk, and experiencing the BPD patient as intentionally manipulative and attention-seeking. Similarly, SUD clinicians may believe that patients choose to be irresponsible with substance use and choose to harm others by patterns of substance use that also include recurrent lying, criminal acts, and violent behavior. In addition to clinician stigma, access-to-care barriers are prominent in both BPD and SUD populations, mostly because of lack of health care insurance.

Two main strategies will improve your capacity to provide clinical care competently and confidently. First, understand the neurobiological underpinnings of symptom expression for both BPD (Iskric and Barkley-Levenson 2021) and SUDs (Koob and Volkow 2016; Kozak et al. 2019). In simplest terms, it is helpful to consider 1) interpersonal hypersensitivity (IHS) as the neurobiological vulnerability leading to BPD presentations of either hyperarousal with behavioral dysregulation or perceived criticism/rejection with highly avoidant behavior, and 2) impulsivity as the neurobiological vulnerability associated with patterns of substance misuse and SUDs. Once the clinician appreciates these vulnerabilities, behavioral presentations may be interpreted as data that provide information about the patient's current state within the illness. For instance, it is helpful to educate colleagues, patients, and families that lying is an indicator of active substance use, in the same way that having a fever may reflect an acute infection. When a person is well and in remission from SUD, lying typically disappears. Similarly, when a BPD patient presents with hostility or avoidance, frequently it is a response to a misperceived threat. If one can elicit what is feared and address it, the response may soften enough to better tolerate and engage in care.

For both BPD and SUDs, predictability is very helpful in structuring care. Aim to be consistent, caring, and responsive rather than reactive, and use clear directives with any care that is prescriptive. The use of a consistent, structured check-in (key questions addressing health safety and target symptoms) at the beginning of each session has several advantages. First, it trains patients in self-assessment, since they know that every session will begin with specific questions about their personal symptom profile and their health safety. Second, it quickly covers the clinical data of highest risk management need, useful for documentation. Third, it facilitates prioritization of the patient session so that time management addresses the greatest risk needs. Fourth, it provides the patient with a consistent expectation of how to enter treatment each session and what you will be looking at together.

The check-in is explained transparently as part of the treatment plan, so that patients understand the rationale and the utility in promoting health and safety. Patients can also appreciate that as they progress in wellness, more time will be available to address quality-of-life goals. The selection of check-in items needs to be personalized, but a general outline includes the following:

> I will ask you to check in at the beginning of every session to tell me about your thoughts and behaviors since we last met. This is so that we always start with the symptoms that pose the greatest safety risk to you. Here is what I would like you to check in on: 1) Have you had suicide thoughts or self-harm behaviors? If yes, describe very briefly. 2) Have you used substances? If yes, describe how often, how much, and any consequences; if no, did you have any urges/cravings or close call situations? 3) Have you taken all your medications exactly as prescribed? Did you miss any? Have you had any side effects? 4) Did you have any dangerous situations I should know about? (This may be personalized to relationships or other disclosed problematic behaviors such as promiscuity, gambling, overspending, etc.)

A check-in should be brief if conducted verbally, no more than 5 minutes, or it may be written up by the patient for your review in-office, depending on what system fits best with your clinical care workflow. The check-in will guide your clinical interventions, and these are best presented to the patient as interventions to promote health and safety, with clear recommendations and rationale. Patients will hold the choice to accept or decline your recommendations except in true emergency situations. Documentation that clearly advised, informed consent was provided, followed by the patient declining recommended treatment, suffices as protective evidence that you delivered current standard of care, which the patient understood but had capacity and autonomy to decline.

Co-occurring Tobacco and Cannabis Use or Other Drug Use Disorders

Many patients with BPD+AUD have other co-occurring substance misuse, particularly prescription medication misuse, tobacco use, cannabis use, and other drug use disorders. We consider these briefly below.

Prescription Medication Misuse and Use Disorder

Four main strategies reduce the risk of prescription medication misuse and addiction.

1. Educate the patient about medication abuse liability during informed consent and agree that the medication trial will be fixed dosing only (no "as needed" dosing and no missed doses). Clarify if this will be a brief-duration trial for acute symptom need (30 days or fewer) or a maintenance augmentation strategy. Make expectations clear; provide standard patient education handouts for all new medications prescribed.
2. Check your state prescription drug monitoring program before prescribing.
3. Prescribe short-duration quantities without refills and assess safety and effectiveness before refilling.
4. Monitor disposal of all discontinued or unused medications.

Tobacco Use

Patients with mental health disorders are the most vulnerable population for nicotine use disorder, and quitting smoking can add 10 years to life expectancy and good health. Smoking cessation is therefore always recommended; treatment should be initiated with a medication (varenicline, combined nicotine replacement therapy, or bupropion) plus counseling to assist a quit attempt (Rigotti et al. 2022). Smoking cessation also improves the probability of promoting alcohol and drug abstinence but may need greater emphasis and support services in substance-using populations (Iyahen et al. 2023). With free tools online, including text message and phone coaching options, patients and clinicians are well equipped to provide smoking cessation interventions (visit https://smokefree.gov/ for assistance). For many, smoking cessation is an iterative process: multiple attempts are the norm. Stay patient and encouraging.

Cannabis Use

Cannabis maintains illegal drug status at the U.S. federal level, but as of June 2024, only four states (Idaho, Kansas, South Carolina, and Wyoming) remain with cannabis in a "fully illegal" status. The remainder have approved medicinal use options or fully legalized status (DISA Global Solutions 2024). On May 21, 2024, the Drug Enforcement Administration proposed that cannabis be rescheduled from its current status (Schedule I controlled substance) to Schedule III, which would better align state and federal regulations.

There are many forms of cannabis for recreational use, and the most dangerous products are those with very high concentrations of Δ9-tetrahydrocannabinol (THC), the main psychoactive component of cannabis products, associated with risk for the developing adolescent brain and for onset of psychosis (Hill et al., 2022). Currently, there is no evidence to support the use of cannabis, medical cannabinoids (nabilone, dronabinol), or cannabidiol in patients with mental health disorders. Therefore, patients should be advised to stop use; those choosing to continue use need to be monitored for signs of psychosis and worsened anxiety or depression. There are no FDA-approved medications to treat cannabis use disorder (CUD). Although cognitive-behavioral therapy is the evidence-based treatment for CUD, sustained abstinence outcomes are notoriously low, and harm-reduction interventions apply (avoiding driving while high, set treatment goals to reduce use, or switch products to lower THC amount).

Other Drug Misuse and Drug Use Disorders

Stimulant drugs (cocaine, methamphetamine) and opioids (fentanyl, heroin) are commonly misused and highly addictive. These drugs may be smoked, insufflated (intranasal), or used intravenously; all routes result in rapid intoxication, and dangerousness is dose dependent. Fentanyl is the opioid with the highest potency to cause respiratory depression and may be lethal in very small doses. There are no medications approved by the FDA for stimulant use disorder, although combining high-dose bupropion with naltrexone shows some efficacy in randomized controlled trials (Trivedi et al. 2021). Three FDA-approved medications to treat opioid use disorder (MOUD) bind and influence the activity of central μ opioid receptors: methadone, a full agonist; buprenorphine, a partial agonist; and naltrexone, an antagonist. Currently buprenorphine and naltrexone may be administered in office-based practices, whereas methadone to treat OUD may be administered only in a federally regulated opioid treatment program (methadone clinic). All three medications have proven efficacy when a patient is adherent to care; overdose risk with opioid relapse is high with patient nonadherence (Burns et al., 2022). MOUD treatment currently recommends long-term maintenance to address the persistent lifetime risk for death by overdose. All patients with OUD should be given a clear recommendation for MOUD as well as naloxone rescue education (naloxone is a potent antagonist that can reverse opioid overdose), training, and access, such as a prescription for nasal Narcan or referral for over-the-counter naloxone (https://narcan.com/).

Training resources for treatment of SUDs are highly recommended. The Provider's Clinical Support System provides free training options to clinicians (https://pcssnow.org/courses/), and the Substance Abuse and Mental Health Services Administration (SAMHSA) offers many options for mental health and substance use disorder training (https://www.samhsa.gov/practitioner-training). The American Society for Addiction Medicine (ASAM) also provides treatment guidelines and extensive training courses in treatment of patients with SUDs (https://www.asam.org/asam-criteria/training-consulting).

Telepsychiatry and SUD Telehealth

Although there are no studies of telehealth treatment of BPD+AUD, there is some evidence for telehealth in BPD (Hudon et al. 2022) and a larger body of evidence for telehealth in SUDs and tobacco cessation (Sweeney et al. 2022). Telehealth treatment is optimal for patients who have successfully engaged in a stabilization treatment where the ability to have hybrid services (some in person, some remotely) may promote treatment adherence and efficiency by its flexibility to patient needs and work-life demands. Whenever engaging in telehealth care, clinicians must know their state requirements in addition to federal requirements, and one should always have the patient's exact location and full address documented before the session proceeds in case one needs to respond immediately to an emergency, such as a suicide attempt or substance poisoning.

Assessment of Risk and Level of Care

Assessing risk for unintentional and intentional injury in BPD and SUDs is central to providing timely interventions to mitigate risk and to improve outcomes. In both BPD and SUDs, a central tenet of treatment is for patients to learn how to experience unhealthy or dangerous thoughts without acting on them. The first thing a patient needs to learn is that it is possible to live with recurrent "relapse thoughts" and to yet maintain safe, healthy behaviors, and indeed many in recovery do exactly that. The second thing to learn together is the exact profile of a patient's personal symptom pattern, colloquially referred to in 12-step programs as "people, places, and things," that elevate risk and occurrence of relapse thoughts. This is critical to identifying early triggers, avoiding high-risk environments when possible, and developing an effective safety plan to keep risk low or to swiftly protect and mitigate risk when warning signs are observed. See Figure 10–1 for a longitudinal schematic of safety planning and patient engagement for mental health and SUDs, including BPD+AUD.

Patient engagement involves the patient taking agency for risk mitigation according to a carefully designed collaborative set of strategies that the clinician and patient develop and refine over time. It is important to recognize and emphasize that strategies must be personalized to work effectively. There are common categories of strategy patients may consider. One is observing a thought and considering why it may have occurred, but keeping the unhealthy thoughts separated from willful or impulsive action. In BPD treatment, this skill may be called "suspending judgment" or "accepting without acting," and in SUD treatment, it may be called "surfing the craving" or labeling the thought "relapse thinking." The idea is to discern intrusive and unhealthy thoughts from rational, healthy thoughts and avoid treating unhealthy thoughts as a directive for action.

Once a patient understands the need to pause and consider, then a recovery action needs to be selected. This piece is very personalized, because for some, meditation is calming, and for others, meditation is agitating; some people need to be alone, and others need to connect for calming; for some, physical exercise is distracting, and for others a hot bath or getting lost in a videogame may be needed. The key is to discover the skills that allow a patient to switch cognitive sets quickly and effectively, the skills that best compete with troubling thoughts or emotional states that elevate risk, and the activities that are mutually exclusive to the risk state (Table 10–1). Patients need to be willing to try lots of new skills and to practice until they have a package of skills that are well suited to their personal temperament and circumstances.

Clinicians need honest data from patients to assess level of risk and potential need for level of care (LOC) change. For both BPD and SUDs, assessment considers symptom frequency, level of intrusiveness, symptom intensity, and symptom or episode duration. The greater the symp-

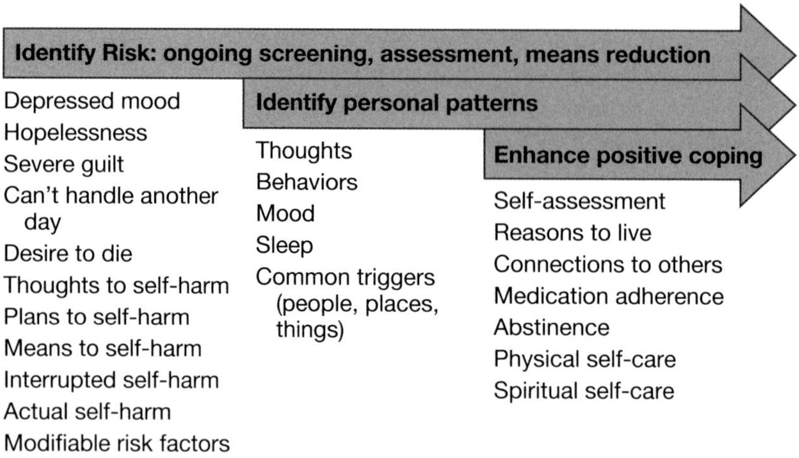

Identify Risk: ongoing screening, assessment, means reduction

Depressed mood
Hopelessness
Severe guilt
Can't handle another day
Desire to die
Thoughts to self-harm
Plans to self-harm
Means to self-harm
Interrupted self-harm
Actual self-harm
Modifiable risk factors

Identify personal patterns

Thoughts
Behaviors
Mood
Sleep
Common triggers (people, places, things)

Enhance positive coping

Self-assessment
Reasons to live
Connections to others
Medication adherence
Abstinence
Physical self-care
Spiritual self-care

Figure 10–1. Longitudinal safety planning and patient engagement for self-injury, suicide, and substance use risks.

Source. L.W. Choi-Kain.

Table 10–1. Personalized safety planning: patient engagement

1. Patient-specific warning signs
2. Who can support you, and how?
3. What can you do to reduce risk, and what are you willing to do?
4. Written pocket reminder
5. Collateral data connections—engage in risk management
6. Medications that target risk factors
7. Peer supports linkage
8. Caring outreach contacts (personal follow-up)
9. Stanley-Brown safety plan: https://suicidesafetyplan.com/training/

Source. L.W. Choi-Kain.

tom intrusiveness, the greater the patient experience of losing control. Risk is highest when symptom intrusiveness, intensity, and episode duration are all reported as severe, especially if symptoms impair sleep health, which adds to risk for self-harm and substance use. When this occurs, a thorough safety assessment is warranted to determine any changes needed to the safety plan or to LOC.

If a change in LOC is not warranted or clinical judgment determines that an LOC change may pose more harm than good, but symptoms are nonetheless severe, the social/community safety net must be strengthened such that the patient is willing to allow supporting people to appreciate the elevated risk and participate in risk mitigation efforts. Means reduction is also essential, and for BPD + SUD patients, it includes working with the patient and social supports to maintain a substance-free environment and to secure any medications that may be lethal in an overdose attempt. It is always important to clearly document how foreseeable risk was assessed, the options that were considered to mitigate risk, and the rationale for options selected to mitigate risk.

Although risk episodes are stressful for patients, families, and clinicians, anticipatory planning for management of risk significantly helps to ease in-the-moment decision-making between patients and the care team and facilitates timely interventions. As patients and clinicians gain experience moving successfully through risk episodes, enduring improvements become more "real" and rewarding for both, supporting good outcomes.

11

Case Example

Lois W. Choi-Kain, M.D., M.Ed.
Carl Fleisher, M.D.

The following clinical vignette illustrates how to apply good psychiatric management of borderline personality disorder and alcohol use disorder (GPM-AUD) principles in common clinical scenarios. We offer **Decision Points** to give readers a chance to think through how they personally would respond before reading further. Afterward, a nonexhaustive list of **Alternative Responses** to the Decision Points are offered for the reader's consideration. To help the reader understand which responses are more or less aligned with the GPM-AUD approach, the reader can rate which responses are helpful (scored as **1**), possibly helpful but with continuing reservations (because it depends on other considerations or because the response's effect seems unpredictable; scored as **2**); and not helpful—or even harmful (scored as **3**).

We encourage readers to think first about what they would do and why and reflect on their reactions to the different alternative responses. The spirit of GPM encourages clinicians to preserve their capacity to think independently and make reasoned decisions in realistically complex clinical situations where no one right answer exists. Rather, we emphasize that good clinical judgment will depend on being aware of why you would take one course of action over another.

The **Discussion** at the end examines the upsides and downsides of each Alternative Response from the GPM-AUD perspective, pointing readers toward relevant sections of the manual where relevant GPM-

AUD principles are presented. Most clinical decisions leave professionals in unresolved dilemmas that they can manage steadily using a coherent set of principles. You might disagree with suggested interventions. We encourage readers to take a position, understand how much it aligns with standards of care and evidence, and identify what GPM-AUD intervention would look like.

At the decision points, choose: 1 = helpful; 2 = possibly helpful, with continuing reservations; 3 = not helpful—or even harmful.

This clinical vignette (which illustrates Chapters 2 ["Overall Principles"], 3 ["Integrating DDP and GPM"], 4 ["Making the Diagnosis"], 5 ["Setting the Framework"], 6 ["Managing Suicidality and Nonsuicidal Self-Injury], 7 ["Pharmacotherapy"], 8 ["Multimodal Treatments"), and 9 ["Levels of Care"]) depicts the case of Belinda, who has both borderline personality disorder (BPD) and alcohol use disorder (AUD), among other psychiatric co-occurring conditions. It illustrates common treatment impasses that can occur with intermittent partially successful treatments for either disorder without an integrated approach to care focused on BPD+AUD. This case example demonstrates the way that diagnostic disclosure and psychoeducation can frame a reorientation to a treatment that is not working, create a new treatment framework to treat BPD and AUD simultaneously, re-establish alliances, and return responsibility to patients for managing their interpersonal and stress sensitivity in a way that promotes support and self-esteem.

Case Vignette: Belinda

Belinda is a 35-year-old woman with two prior hospitalizations for depression and suicidal thoughts, one prior admission to alcohol detoxification with 28-day rehabilitation program, and a long history of ineffective talk therapy with seven different therapists. She currently lives with roommates; is an assistant to a music executive, where she works erratic hours; and attends numerous social functions where alcohol and other drugs are provided. Belinda said that past participation in dialectical behavior therapy (DBT) was helpful for suicidality/self-harm, but she was not able to continue the groups and appointments because of her unpredictable work schedule. She was told by prior therapists that her trauma and emotional dysregulation causes her self-harming behaviors and suicidality, but she has never received a diagnosis of BPD. Her medical history is unremarkable except for hepatitis C, contracted from sexual activity. She has other psychiatric problems, including anxiety, depression, ADHD, and mixed eating disorder. Belinda is referred to you by a colleague who heard you had training in GPM-AUD and felt Belinda would be better off with a different prescribing psychiatrist.

Decision Point 1

In response to your colleague's referral:

A. You tell the colleague that Belinda should go to a residential treatment program for BPD where they will treat her BPD and she can get some sobriety.

B. You accept the opportunity to evaluate Belinda, telling your colleague that you will need a release of information to enable you two to talk and coordinate her care. You and Belinda will decide together that a change in treatment is indicated.

C. You ask your colleague what the problem is in the care and if you can supervise them instead of taking the case.

D. You evaluate the medication regimen and start gabapentin.

You meet with Belinda, who has signed releases for you to speak to the referring clinician. In reviewing her treatment history, Belinda tells you she has sporadically attended AA but has had ups and downs when she has gotten romantically involved with people she meets there, and this causes her to avoid or feel self-conscious when she does attend, worried she will run into someone with whom she has a history. She is currently not in therapy, and tells you she has been there and done that to no benefit. She has been in both cognitive-behavioral and psychodynamic treatments but cannot remember the names of her clinicians. Your colleague, a long-standing psychiatrist who she trusts, has trialed many pharmacologic interventions, although Belinda cannot remember the target problems for which the medications were prescribed. At times, she takes no medication, but has been on SSRIs (e.g., citalopram 40 mg, fluoxetine 20 mg, sertraline 100 mg). Belinda didn't tolerate the medication because of sexual side effects but thought they were partially effective for anxiety/depressive symptoms but not for lability and cravings. She has tried aripiprazole 5 mg daily but stopped taking it because of weight gain. She also tried lamotrigine 200 mg daily, well tolerated, but kept forgetting it some days, so her prescriber stopped it out of worry about her consistency. The one medication she finds consistently helpful is guanfacine ER 4 mg qhs for ADHD; her provider noted that it provided partial benefit and was well tolerated with good adherence. She sometimes takes trazodone 50–100 mg qhs prn for insomnia, which has been moderately effective. When asked about naltrexone, Belinda says her doctor once prescribed it for treating her self-harm at 50 mg daily, but she did not think it worked for her cutting so she stopped taking it. Belinda also has a supply of lorazepam 1 mg, which she takes most days for anxiety.

Decision Point 2

In your first meeting with Belinda:

A. You evaluate Belinda's suicidal and self-harming urges to determine her safety.

B. You tell Belinda that your colleague, her long-standing psychiatrist, has referred her to you for more integrated treatment of her multiple diagnoses. You tell her you are interested in hearing what she thinks is going well, not so well, and what she wants from treatment, so that you can be most prepared to be her ally in the treatment process.

C. You ask Belinda what she sees as her major important psychiatric problems and how they interfere with sustaining or attaining things she wants in life.

D. You tell Belinda she needs to stop taking lorazepam as soon as possible.

You ask Belinda to tell you more about what she most wants to focus on in her psychiatric problems. Belinda starts by telling you that she works hard in all she does but screws up her life all the time with her drinking. She describes having an exciting lifestyle working in the music industry, but she feels very lonely and worries that no one cares about her. Belinda works long hours with little structure, on evenings, weekends, and holidays, waiting for her boss to call or text with tasks and directions. Belinda describes meeting many people in her work that at first she feels optimistic about, but later after socializing, usually in contexts involving drugs or alcohol, she invariably does or says something that she feels embarrassed and ashamed of later, causing her anxiety whenever she has to see the same people in a professional context. She tells you she has had sexual involvements with many colleagues, which is both exciting and regrettable for her. Belinda feels special when it is happening, but later she feels ashamed for her reputation of being promiscuous. She fears that others in the office hate her, since she is aware they gossip about her, and she often lashes out when she perceives they are making fun of her. Burying herself in work helps her avoid her socially troubling interactions, and her boss's dependence on her makes her feel important. Belinda isn't sure what to do about her situation, so she avoids thinking about it by drinking when alone and vaping at night before bedtime.

Belinda says she knows she would be better off sober and asks you if you think she should start going to AA again.

Decision Point 3

In response to Belinda:

A. You tell Belinda she needs to start looking for meetings immediately and get a sponsor.
B. You tell her that despite her high level of functioning, you see that she has a very common form of interpersonal hypersensitivity that can cause major ups and downs in mood, behavior, ways of relating to others, and self-esteem. Ask her if she has heard of the diagnosis of BPD, which reflects this kind of interpersonal hypersensitivity.
C. You tell her she has complex PTSD and needs exposure therapy.
D. You ask about her alcohol and other substance use history and current patterns.

> She readily accepts the diagnosis of BPD and feels it explains why she has so many problems. Belinda tells you she knows her neediness and people-pleasing keeps her on a roller coaster emotionally. She also reflects on how she ends up lashing out at people she wants approval from, which is clearly self-defeating. Belinda says you are the best doctor to ever help her, and that now she feels confident she will get her act together.

Decision Point 4

In response to Belinda's rapid acceptance of the BPD diagnosis and interest in working with you:

A. You immediately shake hands and say you think she will get better now that she knows she has BPD.
B. You tell Belinda that once her BPD is treated, she will definitely not need to use alcohol or substances.
C. You express concerns about the alcohol use, and occasional cannabis use, providing psychoeducation that BPD combines with these substance use problems to amplify problems, with a high addictive reinforcing potential and a loss of control. Inquire about her history of use and current pattern of usage.
D. You talk to her family to see if they know of any childhood traumas she has no memory of currently to rule out complex PTSD.

> Belinda tells you her alcohol use started at 14 years old. Currently, she drinks a shot of vodka daily around 10 am and before going to bed, with two to four drinks throughout the day, depending on the meals and social events her work involves. She has had a number of minor car accidents

and has embarrassed herself in front of her boss and his clients on a number of occasions, but her boss tolerates her intoxication because he thinks it is funny and cute. Her other substance use includes vaping marijuana on her nights off. When asked about the reasons she uses alcohol, Belinda says she drinks to cope with feeling numb/empty and with being overwhelmed. In sober moments, she feels shame that her excessive drinking reinforces or exacerbates rejection sensitivity. Self-harm doesn't occur by itself, rather it typically follows drinking. In one episode, after drinking, she cut herself on her cheek and texted a picture to an ex-partner in a bid to get back together. Belinda attempted to join AA, but her interpersonal hypersensitivity led to perceived rejection by sponsors and a few sexual encounters with other AA participants, followed by gradual withdrawal from participation in the 12-step group.

Decision Point 5

In response to her report:

A. You say to definitely stop using substances; they cause you to do things you will regret. Provide you-can-do-it encouragement.
B. You explore the pros and cons of using alcohol and cannabis using motivational interviewing.
C. You ask what goals she has related to her substance use problems.
D. You have her call a different 28-day program than she went to, because one that focuses on DBT and sobriety will help her more than the one she attended.

You work with Belinda on her dialectical consideration of why she uses alcohol throughout the day. She starts to talk about her interpersonal interactions and her thoughts about her worth, which rises and falls throughout the day. Belinda describes that she feels a bit of a boost from the alcohol at first, which propels her work throughout the day, and if she is feeling anxious or sad, it takes the edge off of that. You discuss the interpersonal hypersensitivity model and how it relates to her BPD symptoms and alcohol use. For the time being, she does not feel the vaping is a problem.

Decision Point 6

As a next step:

A. You insist on her cutting down on vaping at the same time as alcohol.
B. You ask her about what her personal goals are for her occupation. Discuss what she likes and does not like about her current job, eval-

uating whether it is a source of undue exposure to interpersonal stressors.

C. You call her family to set up an appointment to plan an intervention.

D. You discuss starting naltrexone to help her diminish the priming effects of alcohol to make it easier for her to stop drinking when she starts and to cut down urges.

Belinda agrees to start naltrexone and is thoughtful about the benefits and drawbacks of her current work situation. She wonders whether her accumulated reputation is something she can ever overcome. With your advisement about what to say, she tells her boss she needs a more predictable schedule to take better care of herself, acknowledging her erratic behaviors in the office. He agrees temporarily to see how this works for him. Belinda begins to cut down her alcohol use, no longer drinking in the morning or at bedtime. One month into treatment, Belinda's boss tells her she is being terminated, because he really needs someone who can cater to his round-the-clock schedule. Belinda maturely agrees to move on, but then feels lost and relapses to both drinking and self-harm. She calls you telling you she can't do this, that she has consumed four shots of vodka, and that she's going to think by the bridge, and she hangs up. She does not call back when you try to reach her.

Decision Point 7

In response:

A. You leave Belinda a message and ask her to call you back, telling her you can't help her if you can't discuss more about her current problem, emphasizing you really want to lean into this problem rather than avoid it.

B. You text her to use her safety plan.

C. You call 911 to have a safety check at her apartment.

D. You call a 28-day treatment facility to hold a bed.

Belinda calls you back and agrees to go into the hospital for stabilization. She does not require detoxification, but she thinks that given her lack of structure and support, she does want to go to a brief intensive outpatient program to have daily contact with others. You counsel her on use of AA and the pitfalls of interpersonal hypersensitivity, as a way to frame the rules and roles of AA as a good opportunity to socialize herself to AA's culture in a more steady way than her prior experience. Belinda starts sharing more at AA, makes friends, gets a sponsor, and engages in step work. In her free time, she looks for a job she can do temporarily for structure while she sorts out her next steps. Belinda sees you once a week, goes to AA, and starts meeting up with sober friends she has not seen because of the demands of her prior job. She stops using alcohol, but vapes on the weekend. Belinda's BPD improves, although she is still insecure in relation to her sponsor and certain friends, but she uses your time together to understand and strategize how to manage her vulnerabilities.

Discussion

1. In response to your colleague's referral:

   A. You tell the colleague that Belinda should go to a residential treatment program for BPD where they will treat her BPD and she can get some sobriety.

      [Score 3] Training sometimes leads us to reflexively match treatments to diagnosis without consideration of readiness, capacity to maintain a lower level of care, and life structures that would be disrupted by inpatient or residential treatment. Understanding the ASAM guidelines will teach clinicians that sending patients to a higher level of care than indicated can be harmful. Evaluating the patient's problems, stability level, and motivation is required before recommending intensive levels of treatment (Chapter 9).

   B. You accept the opportunity to evaluate Belinda, telling your colleague that you will need a release of information to enable you two to talk and coordinate her care. You and Belinda will decide together that a change in treatment is indicated.

      [Score 1] This allows you to meet and decide collaboratively with Belinda. She will need to decide whether you would be helpful (Chapter 3). Gathering information from her long-standing treater can enhance your understanding of the situation.

   C. You ask your colleague what the problem is in the care and if you can supervise them instead of taking the case.

      [Score 2] This choice may be indicated if the patient is too attached to this treater to switch to another one. Providing a GPM-AUD framework to a professional who both knows the patient well and maintains a good alliance is worth preserving in some cases if they are willing and able to spend the time learning. In other cases, transfer with the prior clinician's support may be more practical.

D. You evaluate the medication regimen and start gabapentin.

[Score 3] This choice sets a problematic focus on medications or nonpsychologically oriented, passively received solutions to complex personality and substance use or behavioral tendencies. This might be indicated later, but jumping to a concrete solution before building a narrative also is not recommended since emotional processing of experience and building narratives is central to recovery in treatment of AUD and BPD (Chapter 3). This maneuver would not allow you and the patient to "think first" (Chapter 2).

2. In your first meeting with Belinda:

A. You evaluate Belinda's suicidal and self-harming urges to determine her safety.

[Score 2] Because Belinda's self-harm is currently not active, prioritizing that as a focus may miss the opportunity for gaining a larger context in which to understand broader BPD and AUD symptoms. At the end of the first appointment, if indicated, inquiring about current urges and a safety plan is appropriate and may require a follow-up to complete.

B. You tell Belinda that your colleague, her long-standing psychiatrist, has referred her to you for more integrated treatment of her multiple diagnoses. You tell her you are interested in hearing what she thinks is going well, not so well, and what she wants from treatment, so that you can be most prepared to be her ally in the treatment process.

[Score 1] This choice shows the patient that her understanding of her problem is important and sets the stage for her to have more ownership of both her problems and treatment. This also puts her in the driver's seat of charting the narrative of what isn't going optimally in life to support her self-esteem and agency.

C. You ask Belinda what she sees as her major important psychiatric problems and how they interfere with sustaining or attaining things she wants in life.

[Score 1] Belinda has multiple psychiatric concerns, but focusing on what she finds most problematic at the initiation of treatment will enable you to set a framework to focus on BPD and AUD primarily, and evaluate other diagnoses over time in the initial months of treatment.

D. You tell Belinda she needs to stop taking lorazepam as soon as possible.

[**Score 3**] This maneuver requires a more collaborative approach where psychoeducation provides an opportunity to inform not advise (Chapter 3). Taking time to understand how she is using lorazepam, determining whether or not she finds it helpful, and providing psychoeducation about its contribution to disinhibition may win her motivation to stop rather than it being imposed on her.

3. In response to Belinda:

A. You tell Belinda she needs to start looking for meetings immediately and get a sponsor.

[**Score 3**] More evaluation is needed to help her understand the treatment recommendation of AA to frame how she can use it optimally. Because AA did not work for her before, helping her understand its role and function may help her orient to it differently (Chapter 8).

B. You tell her that despite her high level of functioning, you see that she has a very common form of interpersonal hypersensitivity that can cause major ups and downs in mood, behavior, ways of relating to others, and self-esteem. Ask her if she has heard of the diagnosis of BPD, which reflects this kind of interpersonal hypersensitivity.

[**Score 1**] This choice ties her interpersonal problems to her vulnerability to fluctuations in moods and ingratiating self-sacrificing behavior to angry confrontation (Chapter 2).

C. You tell her she has complex PTSD and needs exposure therapy.

[**Score 3**] Belinda has not provided any cause for considering PTSD. Evaluate her psychiatric and social history more thoroughly first.

D. You ask her about her alcohol and other substance use history and current patterns.

[**Score 1**] Put substance use at the forefront with BPD as the central focus to stabilize her situation and treatment first, to provide a better platform for using treatment for any disorder (Chapter 1).

4. In response to Belinda's rapid acceptance of the BPD diagnosis and interest in working with you:

A. You immediately shake hands and say you think she will get better now that she knows she has BPD.

[**Score 3**] Recovery is a difficult process, and being realistic about the challenges and taking neutrality to allow her greater ownership are indicated (Chapters 3 and 8).

B. You tell Belinda that once her BPD is treated, she will definitely not need to use alcohol or substances.

[**Score 3**] Psychoeducation about interactions between BPD and AUD are helpful, including ongoing susceptibility to a unique reaction and functions of alcohol use in BPD (Chapter 4).

C. You express concerns about the alcohol use and occasional cannabis use, providing psychoeducation that BPD combines with these substance use problems to amplify problems, with a high addictive reinforcing potential and a loss of control. Inquire about her history of use and current pattern of usage.

[**Score 1**] Providing psychoeducation about substance use in BPD as well as the interference of alcohol use on emotional processing as part of the psychotherapeutic treatment helps the patient understand why sobriety is important to the goals of treatment for her BPD (Chapter 4).

D. You talk to her family to see if they know of any childhood traumas she has no memory of currently to rule out complex PTSD.

[**Score 3**] Enlisting family in the process without permission or collaboration by the patient may undermine her agency and make her an object of criticism rather than an agent in taking control of her own life with space to reflect, process, and think (Chapter 3).

5. In response to her report:

A. You say to definitely stop using substances, they cause you to do things you will regret. Provide you-can-do-it encouragement.

[**Score 3**] While this may seem self-evident, making more space for her to be broader in her thinking to reduce splitting and ambivalence will stabilize changes to be less superficial.

B. You explore the pros and cons of using alcohol and cannabis using motivational interviewing.

[**Score 1**] Motivational interviewing enables the patient to own both the drawbacks of using and the reasons to stop to fuel her decision step by step to not use (Chapter 4).

C. You ask what goals she has related to her substance use problems.

[**Score 1**] Goal setting is an important part of getting started in GPM to organize a collaborative working alliance and evaluating the value of the treatment according to how well it is meeting goals, rather than an unstructured subjective sense of connectedness (Chapter 5).

D. You have her call a different 28-day program than she went to, because one that focuses on DBT and sobriety will help her more than the one she attended.

[**Score 3**] Clinicians can use ASAM guidelines to assess level of care best suited for her current severity of substance use risk (Chapter 9).

6. As a next step:

A. You insist on her cutting down on vaping at the same time as alcohol.

[**Score 3**] Belinda and you have not really yet fully understood vaping, which might function similarly to alcohol, but doubling the responsibility on the patient to manage ambitious goals may inadvertently undermine self-esteem and motivation. Setting goals is a stepwise process and must be centered on the patient's valued outcomes rather than the clinician who can only inform, not advise (Chapters 3 and 5).

B. You ask her about what her personal goals are for her occupation. Discuss what she likes and does not like about her current job, evaluating whether it is a source of undue exposure to interpersonal stressors.

[**Score 1**] Understanding her problems in the larger context of her work, self-direction, and identity is a part of the developmental support for repairing part of her personality dysfunction. Situational changes can relieve drivers of symptom oscillations for BPD, and the exposure to substances in her current job context may make it difficult for her to reach her goals. Providing a judgment-free zone to contemplate this issue is likely to help her think about whether this current job is helping her meet her ultimate goals (Chapters 3 and 5).

C. You call her family to set up an appointment to plan an intervention.

[**Score 3**] While family involvement is helpful, calling them without proper collaboration, understanding, and psychoeducation may not serve in the ultimate goal of creating a more support-ive social safety net for Belinda. Evaluate with her and with your own conversation with them what is needed, first in terms of psychoeducation, and then in terms of support for them to learn how to best contribute to the ultimate goals of aiding Belinda's treatment rather than forcing behavioral change (Chapter 8).

D. You discuss starting naltrexone to help her diminish the priming effects of alcohol to make it easier for her to stop drinking when she starts and to cut down on urges.

[**Score 1**] This is a good idea. Effective treatment for reducing drivers of alcohol use should be integrated into the overall picture of care. Naltrexone is easily administered, well tolerated, and effective. Psychoeducation about its benefits will help Belinda best understand how to use it—its effectiveness will be determined by her use of it (Chapter 7).

7. In response:

A. You leave Belinda a message and ask her to call you back, telling her you can't help her if you can't discuss more about her current problem, emphasizing you really want to lean into this problem rather than avoid it.

[**Score 1**] Communicate in whatever way you can that you need her to discuss with you how the two of you can work together through this crisis. Lean into her fight and flight, as her life structure is realistically threatened. If you can balance leaning in without taking over, her agency and chance to make a decision with your help about how to manage is optimal (Chapter 2 and 6).

B. You text her to use her safety plan.

[**Score 2**] It is up to Belinda to use an established safety plan, but asking her to be more communicative about what is going on would be ideal.

C. You call 911 to have a safety check at her apartment.

[**Score 2**] If a clinician is truly worried and uneasy about the uncertainty, having an evaluation before deciding next steps is appropriate (Chapter 6).

D. You call a 28-day treatment facility to hold a bed.

[**Score 3**] This is premature without collaboratively assessing the situation (Chapter 9).

12

References

Adler KA, Finch EF, Rodriguez-Villa AM, Choi-Kain LW: Primary care providers, in Applications of Good Psychiatric Management for Borderline Personality Disorder. Edited by Choi-Kain LW, Gunderson JG. Washington, DC, American Psychiatric Association Publishing, 2019, pp 169–186

Agostinelli G, Brown JM, Miller WR: Effects of normative feedback on consumption among heavy drinking college students. J Drug Educ 25(1):31–40, 1995 7776148

Agrawal HR, Gunderson J, Holmes BM, Lyons-Ruth K: Attachment studies with borderline patients: a review. Harv Rev Psychiatry 12(2):94–104, 2004 15204804

Alcoholics Anonymous: Alcoholics Anonymous Big Book, 4th Edition. New York, Alcoholics Anonymous World Services, 2004

American Psychiatric Association: Diagnostic and Statistical Manual of Mental Disorders, 4th Edition. Washington, DC, American Psychiatric Association, 1994

American Psychiatric Association: Diagnostic and Statistical Manual of Mental Disorders, 5th Edition, Text Revision. Washington, DC, American Psychiatric Association, 2022

American Psychiatric Association: The American Psychiatric Association Practice Guideline for the Treatment of Patients With Borderline Personality Disorder. American Psychiatric Association, 2023. Available at: https://www.psychiatry.org/getmedia/3ac9a443-4590-47e6-ad9b-0b2d1cff4d53/APA-Borderline-Personality-Disorder-Practice-Guideline-Under-Copyediting.pdf. Accessed February 20, 2024.

American Psychological Association. APA PsycTests. Available at: https://www.apa.org/pubs/databases/psyctests. Accessed March 4, 2024.

American Society of Addiction Medicine. The ASAM Clinical Practice Guideline on Alcohol Withdrawal Management. ASAM, 2020. Available at: https://www.asam.org/docs/default-source/quality-science/the_asam_clinical_practice_guideline_on_alcohol-1.pdf. Accessed March 19, 2024.

American Society of Addiction Medicine. The ASAM Criteria, 4th Edition. ASAM, 2024. Available at: https://www.asam.org/asam-criteria/asam-criteria-4th-edition. Accessed March 20, 2024.

Anandarajah G, Hight E: Spirituality and medical practice: using the HOPE questions as a practical tool for spiritual assessment. Am Fam Physician 63(1):81–89, 2001 11195773

Andriessen K, Krysinska K, Hill NTM, et al: Effectiveness of interventions for people bereaved through suicide: a systematic review of controlled studies of grief, psychosocial and suicide-related outcomes. BMC Psychiatry 19(1):49, 2019a 30700267

Andriessen K, Krysinska K, Kõlves K, Reavley N: Suicide postvention service models and guidelines 2014–2019: a systematic review. Front Psychol 10:2677, 2019b 31849779

Anton RF, Latham P, Voronin K, et al: Efficacy of gabapentin for the treatment of alcohol use disorder in patients with withdrawal symptoms: a randomized clinical trial. JAMA Intern Med 180(5):728–736, 2020

Anton RF, O'Malley SS, Ciraulo DA, et al; COMBINE Study Research Group: Combined pharmacotherapies and behavioral interventions for alcohol dependence: the COMBINE study: a randomized controlled trial. JAMA 295(17):2003–2017, 2006 16670409

Apodaca TR, Longabaugh R: Mechanisms of change in motivational interviewing: a review and preliminary evaluation of the evidence. Addiction 104(5):705–715, 2009 19413785

The ASAM Clinical Practice Guideline on Alcohol Withdrawal Management. J Addict Med 14(3S Suppl 1):1–72, 2020 32511109

Aviram RB, Brodsky BS, Stanley B: Borderline personality disorder, stigma, and treatment implications. Harv Rev Psychiatry 14(5):249–256, 2006 16990170

Bahji A, Bach P, Danilewitz M, et al: Comparative efficacy and saftey of pharmacotherapies for alcohol withdrawal: a systematic review and network meta-analysis. Addiction (Abingdon, England) 117(10):2591–2601, 2022

Ball SA, Maccarelli LM, LaPaglia DM, Ostrowski MJ: Randomized trial of dual-focused vs. single-focused individual therapy for personality disorders and substance dependence. J Nerv Ment Dis 199(5):319–328, 2011 21543951

Barnicot K, Katsakou C, Marougka S, Priebe S: Treatment completion in psychotherapy for borderline personality disorder: a systematic review and meta-analysis. Acta Psychiatr Scand 123(5):327–338, 2011 21166785

Bateman A, Fonagy P: Mentalization-Based Treatment for Personality Disorders: A Practical Guide. Oxford, UK, Oxford University Press, 2016

Baumeister RF, Leary MR: The need to belong: desire for interpersonal attachments as a fundamental human motivation. Psychol Bull 117(3):497–529, 1995 7777651

Baumeister RF, DeWall CN, Ciarocco NJ, Twenge JM: Social exclusion impairs self-regulation. J Pers Soc Psychol 88(4):589–604, 2005 15796662

Beeney JE, Hallquist MN, Clifton AD, et al: Social disadvantage and borderline personality disorder: a study of social networks. Personal Disord 9(1):62–72, 2018 27936840

Bender DS, Dolan RT, Skodol AE, et al: Treatment utilization by patients with personality disorders. Am J Psychiatry 158(2):295–302, 2001 11156814

Bender DS, Skodol AE, Pagano ME, et al: Prospective assessment of treatment use by patients with personality disorders. Psychiatr Serv 57(2):254–257, 2006 16452705

Bertsch K, Gamer M, Schmidt B, et al: Oxytocin and reduction of social threat hypersensitivity in women with borderline personality disorder. Am J Psychiatry 170(10):1169–1177, 2013 23982273

Besson J, Aeby F, Kasas A, et al: Combined efficacy of acamprosate and disulfiram in the treatment of alcoholism: a controlled study. Alcohol Clin Exp Res 22(3):573–579, 1998 9622434

Bischof G, Bischof A, Rumpf H-J: Motivational interviewing: an evidence-based approach for use in medical practice. Dtsch Arztebl Int 118(7):109–115, 2021 33835006

Black DW, Blum N, Pfohl B, Hale N: Suicidal behavior in borderline personality disorder: prevalence, risk factors, prediction, and prevention. J Pers Disord 18(3):226–239, 2004 15237043

Blodgett JC, Del Re AC, Maisel NC, Finney JW: A meta-analysis of topiramate's effects for individuals with alcohol use disorders. Alcohol (Hanover) 38(6):1481–1488, 2014 24796492

Bohnert ASB, Ilgen MA: Understanding links among opioid use, overdose, and suicide. N Engl J Med 380(1):71–79, 2019 30601750

Bohus M, Kleindienst N, Limberger MF, et al: The short version of the Borderline Symptom List (BSL-23): development and initial data on psychometric properties. Psychopathology 42(1):32–39, 2009 19023232

Borges G, Walters EE, Kessler RC: Associations of substance use, abuse, and dependence with subsequent suicidal behavior. Am J Epidemiol 151(8):781–789, 2000 10965975

Borges G, Bagge CL, Cherpitel CJ, et al: A meta-analysis of acute use of alcohol and the risk of suicide attempt. Psychol Med 47(5):949–957, 2017 27928972

Bouza C, Angeles M, Muñoz A, Amate JM: Efficacy and safety of naltrexone and acamprosate in the treatment of alcohol dependence: a systematic review. Addiction 99(7):811–828, 2004 15200577

Bradley KA, Bush KR, Epler AJ, et al: Two brief alcohol-screening tests from the Alcohol Use Disorders Identification Test (AUDIT): validation in a female Veterans Affairs patient population. Arch Intern Med 163(7):821–829, 2003

Brañas MJAA, Croci MS, Ravagnani Salto AB, et al: Neuroimaging studies of nonsuicidal self-injury in youth: a systematic review. Life (Basel) 11(8):729, 2021 34440473

Brañas MJAA, Croci MS, Murray GE, Choi-Kain LW: The relationship between self-harm and suicide in adolescents and young adults. Psychiatr Ann 52(8):311–317, 2022

Bresin K, Mekawi Y. Different ways to drown out the pain: a meta-analysis of the association between nonsuicidal self-injury and alcohol use. Arch Suicide Res 26(2):348–369, 2022

Brooks AT, Lòpez MM, Ranucci A, et al: A qualitative exploration of social support during treatment for severe alcohol use disorder and recovery. Addict Behav Rep 6:76–82, 2017 29430516

Brower KJ, Myra Kim H, Strobbe S, et al: A randomized double-blind pilot trial of gabapentin versus placebo to treat alcohol dependence and comorbid insomnia. Alcohol (Hanover) 32(8):1429–1438, 2008 18540923

Burnette EM, Nieto SJ, Grodin EN, et al: Novel agents for the pharmacological treatment of alcohol use disorder. Drugs 82(3):251–274, 2022 35133639

Burns M, Tang L, Chang CH, et al: Duration of medication treatment for opioid-use disorder and risk of overdose among Medicaid enrollees in 11 states: a retrospective cohort study. Addiction 117(12):3079–3088, 2022 35652681

Bush K, Kivlahan DR, McDonell MB, et al; Ambulatory Care Quality Improvement Project: The AUDIT alcohol consumption questions (AUDIT-C): an effective brief screening test for problem drinking. Ambulatory Care Quality Improvement Project (ACQUIP). Alcohol Use Disorders Identification Test. Arch Intern Med 158(16):1789–1795, 1998 9738608

Carpenter RW, Trela CJ, Lane SP, et al: Elevated rate of alcohol consumption in borderline personality disorder patients in daily life. Psychopharmacology 234(22):3395–3406, 2017

Celik M, Gold MS, Fuehrlein B: A narrative review of current and emerging trends in the treatment of alcohol use disorder. Brain Sci 14(3):294, 2024

Center for Motivation and Change: The Parent's 20 Minute Guide, 2nd Edition. 2016a. Lulu.com

Center for Motivation and Change: The Partner's 20 Minute Guide, 2nd Edition. 2016b. Lulu.com

Chanen AM, Jovev M, Djaja D, et al: Screening for borderline personality disorder in outpatient youth. J Pers Disord 22(4):353–364, 2008b 18684049

Chanen AM, Berk M, Thompson K: Integrating early intervention for borderline personality disorder and mood disorders. Harv Rev Psychiatry 24(5):330–341, 2016 27144298

Chesin MS, Jeglic EL, Stanley B: Pathways to high-lethality suicide attempts in individuals with borderline personality disorder. Arch Suicide Res 14(4):342–362, 2010 21082450

Chetty A, Guse T, Malema M: Integrated vs non-integrated treatment outcomes in dual diagnosis disorders: a systematic review. Health SA 28:2094, 2023

Chick J, Lehert P, Landron F; Plinius Maior Society: Does acamprosate improve reduction of drinking as well as aiding abstinence? J Psychopharmacol 17(4):397–402, 2003 14870951

Choi-Kain LW, Gunderson JG: Applications of Good Psychiatric Management for Borderline Personality Disorder. Washington, DC, American Psychiatric Association Publishing, 2019

Choi-Kain LW, Sharp C: Handbook of Good Psychiatric Management for Adolescents With Borderline Personality Disorder. Washington, DC, American Psychiatric Association Publishing, 2021

Choi-Kain LW, Albert EB, Gunderson JG: Evidence-based treatments for borderline personality disorder: implementation, integration, and stepped care. Harv Rev Psychiatry 24(5):342–356, 2016 27603742

Choi-Kain LW, Finch EF, Masland SR, et al: What works in the treatment of borderline personality disorder. Curr Behav Neurosci Rep 4(1):21–30, 2017 28331780

Chugani CD, Byrd AL, Pedersen SL, et al: Affective and sensation-seeking pathways linking borderline personality disorder symptoms and alcohol-related problems in young women. J Pers Disord 34(3):420–431, 2020 30179582

Cloud J: The mystery of borderline personality disorder. Time Magazine, January 8, 2009

Cohen S: Social relationships and health. Am Psychol 59(8):676–684, 2004 15554821

Cohen S, Wills TA: Stress, social support, and the buffering hypothesis. Psychol Bull 98(2):310–357, 1985 3901065

Cohen SM, Alexander RS, Holt SR: The spectrum of alcohol use: epidemiology, diagnosis, and treatment. Med Clin North Am 106(1):43–60, 2022 34823734

Colmenero-Navarrete L, García-Sancho E, Salguero JM: Relationship between emotion regulation and suicide ideation and attempt in adults and adolescents: a systematic review. Arch Suicide Res 26(4):1702–1735, 2022 34821201

Connery HS, Weiss RD, Griffin ML, et al: Suicidal motivations among opioid overdose survivors: replication and extension. Drug Alcohol Depend 235:109437, 2022 35427980

Conrod PJ, Nikolaou K: Annual research review: On the developmental neuropsychology of substance use disorders. J Child Psychol Psychiatry 57(3):371–394, 2016 26889898

Cristea IA, Gentili C, Cotet CD, et al: Efficacy of psychotherapies for borderline personality disorder: a systematic review and meta-analysis. JAMA Psychiatry 74(4):319–328, 2017 28249086

Daros AR, Zakzanis KK, Ruocco AC: Facial emotion recognition in borderline personality disorder. Psychol Med 43(9):1953–1963, 2013 23149223 de Guzman M, Bird G, Banissy MJ, Catmur C. Self other control processes in social cognition: from imitation to empathy. Philos Trans R Soc B Biol Sci 371(1686):20150079, 2016

Devynck F, Rousseau A, Romo L: Does repetitive negative thinking influence alcohol use? A systematic review of the literature. Front Psychol 10(July):1482, 2019 31333536

Dimeff LA, Linehan MM: Dialectical behavior therapy for substance abusers. Addict Sci Clin Pract 4(2):39–47, 2008 18497717

DISA Global Solutions: Marijuana Legality by State. 2024. Available at: https://disa.com/marijuana-legality-by-state/. Accessed March 29, 2024.

Distel MA, Trull TJ, Derom CA, et al: Heritability of borderline personality disorder features is similar across three countries. Psychol Med 38(9):1219–1229, 2008 17988414

Dulit RA, Fyer MR, Haas GL, et al: Substance use in borderline personality disorder. Am J Psychiatry 147(8):1002–1007, 1990 2375433

Edwards AC, Ohlsson H, Sundquist J, et al: Alcohol use disorder and risk of suicide in a Swedish population-based cohort. Am J Psychiatry 177(7):627–634, 2020 32160767

Erikson EH: Growth and crises of the "healthy personality," in Symposium on the Healthy Personality. Edited by Senn MJE. New York, Macy Foundation, 1950, pp 91–146

Esang M, Ahmed S: A closer look at substance use and suicide. Am J Psychiatry Resid J 13(6):6–8, 2018

Ewing JA: Detecting alcoholism: the CAGE questionnaire. JAMA 252(14):1905–1907, 1984 6471323

Favril L, Yu R, Uyar A, et al: Risk factors for suicide in adults: systematic review and meta-analysis of psychological autopsy studies. Evid Based Ment Health 25(4):148–155, 2022 36162975

Fein G, Nip V: Borderline personality symptoms in short-term and long-term abstinent alcohol dependence. Alcohol Clin Exp Res 36(7):1188–1195, 2012

Fertuck EA, Grinband J, Stanley B: Facial trust appraisal negatively biased in borderline personality disorder. Psychiatry Res 207(3):195–202, 2013 23419843

Figueiredo M, Caldeira C, Chen Y, Zheng K: Routine self-tracking of health: reasons, facilitating factors, and the potential impact on health management practices. AMIA Annu Symp Proc 2017:706–714, 2018 29854136

Fineberg SK, Gupta S, Leavitt J: Collaborative deprescribing in borderline personality disorder: a narrative review. Harv Rev Psychiatry 27(2):75–86, 2019 30676404

Flynn S, Graney J, Nyathi T, et al: Clinical characteristics and care pathways of patients with personality disorder who died by suicide. BJPsych Open 6(2):e29, 2020

Fonagy P, Luyten P, Allison E: Epistemic petrification and the restoration of epistemic trust: a new conceptualization of borderline personality disorder and its psychosocial treatment. J Pers Disord 29(5):575–609, 2015a 26393477

Foote J, Wilkens C, Kosanke N, Higgs S: Beyond Addiction: How Science and Kindness Help People Change. New York, Scribner, 2014

Fuller RK, Branchey L, Brightwell DR, et al: Disulfiram treatment of alcoholism: a Veterans Administration cooperative study. JAMA 256(11):1449–1455, 1986 3528541

Furieri FA, Nakamura-Palacios EM: Gabapentin reduces alcohol consumption and craving: a randomized, double-blind, placebo-controlled trial. J Clin Psychiatry 68(11):1691–1700, 2007 18052562

Gabbard GO: An overview of countertransference with borderline patients. J Psychother Pract Res 2(1):7–18, 1993 22700123

Gad MA, Pucker HE, Hein KE, et al: Facets of identity disturbance reported by patients with borderline personality disorder and personality-disordered comparison subjects over 20 years of prospective follow-up. Psychiatry Res 271:76–82, 2019 30469092

Galanter M, White WL, Ziegler PP, Hunter B: An empirical study on the construct of "God" in the Twelve Step process. Am J Drug Alcohol Abuse 46(6):731–738, 2020 32870030

Gianoli MO, Jane JS, O'Brien E, Ralevski E: Treatment for comorbid borderline personality disorder and alcohol use disorders: a review of the evidence and future recommendations. Exp Clin Psychopharmacol 20(4):333–344, 2012 22686496

Giesen-Bloo J, van Dyck R, Spinhoven P, et al: Outpatient psychotherapy for borderline personality disorder: randomized trial of schema-focused therapy vs transference-focused therapy. Arch Gen Psychiatr 63(6):649–658, 2006

Gold LH, Frierson RL; American Psychiatric Association Publishing: The American Psychiatric Association Publishing Textbook of Suicide Risk Assessment and Management, 3rd Edition. Washington, DC, American Psychiatric Association Publishing, 2020

Goldblatt MJ, Ronningstam E, Herbstman B, Schechter M: Therapists' reactions to the suicide of a patient: traumatic loss impairing bereavement and growth. Scand Psychoanal Rev 43(2):78–86, 2020

Goldfried MR: What has psychotherapy inherited from Carl Rogers? Psychotherapy (Chic) 44(3):249–252, 2007 22122246

Goldfried MR: Obtaining consensus in psychotherapy: what holds us back? Am Psychol 74(4):484–496, 2019 30221947

Gomes K, Hart KE: Adherence to recovery practices prescribed by Alcoholics Anonymous: benefits to sustained abstinence and subjective quality of life. Alcohol Treat Q 27(2):223–235, 2009

Goodman M, Tomas IA, Temes CM, et al: Suicide attempts and self-injurious behaviours in adolescent and adult patients with borderline personality disorder. Personal Ment Health 11(3):157–163, 2017 28544496

Gossop M, Keaney F, Stewart D, et al: A Short Alcohol Withdrawal Scale (SAWS): development and psychometric properties. Addict Biol 7(1):37–43, 2002 11900621

Grant BF, Chou SP, Goldstein RB, et al: Prevalence, correlates, disability, and comorbidity of DSM-IV borderline personality disorder: results from the Wave 2 National Epidemiologic Survey on Alcohol and Related Conditions. J Clin Psychiatry 69(4):533–545, 2008 18426259

Grant BF, Goldstein RB, Saha TD, et al: Epidemiology of DSM-5 Alcohol Use Disorder: results From the National Epidemiologic Survey on Alcohol and Related Conditions III. JAMA Psychiatry 72(8):757–766, 2015 26039070

Gratz KL, Roemer L: The relationship between emotion dysregulation and deliberate self-harm among female undergraduate students at an urban commuter university. Cogn Behav Ther 37(1):14–25, 2008 18365795

Greenfield BL, Tonigan JS: The general Alcoholics Anonymous tools of recovery: the adoption of 12-step practices and beliefs. Psychol Addict Behav 27(3):553–561, 2013 22867293

Greenfield SF, Sugarman DE, Freid CM, et al: Group therapy for women with substance use disorders: results from the Women's Recovery Group Study. Drug Alcohol Depend 142:245–253, 2014 25042759

Gregory C, Chorny Y, McLeod SL, Mohindra R: First-line medications for the outpatient treatment of alcohol use disorder: a systematic review of perceived barriers. J Addict Med 16(4):e210–e218, 2022

Gregory RJ: Dynamic deconstructive psychotherapy for substance use disorders co-occurring with personality disorders, in Contemporary Psychodynamic Psychotherapy: Evolving Clinical Practice. Cambridge, MA, Academic Press, 2019, pp 163–175

Gregory RJ: Remediation for Treatment-Resistant Borderline Personality Disorder: Manual of Dynamic Deconstructive Psychotherapy. 2022. Available at: https://www.upstate.edu/psych/pdf/manual-2-14-23.pdf. Accessed February 20, 2024.

Gregory RJ, Mustata GT: Magical thinking in narratives of adolescent cutters. J Adolesc 35(4):1045–1051, 2012 22464283

Gregory RJ, Remen AL: A manual-based psychodynamic therapy for treatment-resistant borderline personality disorder. Psychotherapy (Chic) 45(1):15–27, 2008 22122362

Gregory RJ, Chlebowski S, Kang D, et al: A controlled trial of psychodynamic psychotherapy for co-occurring borderline personality disorder and alcohol use disorder. Psychotherapy (Chic) 45(1):28–41, 2008 22122363

Gregory RJ, DeLucia-Deranja E, Mogle JA: Dynamic deconstructive psychotherapy versus optimized community care for borderline personality disorder co-occurring with alcohol use disorders: a 30-month follow-up. J Nerv Ment Dis 198(4):292–298, 2010 20386259

Gunderson JG: Borderline Personality Disorder, 1st Edition. Washington, DC, American Psychiatric Association Publishing, 1984

Gunderson JG: The borderline patient's intolerance of aloneness: insecure attachments and therapist availability. Am J Psychiatr 153(6):752–758, 1996

Gunderson JG: Borderline Personality Disorder: A Clinical Guide. Washington, DC, American Psychiatric Association Publishing, 2001

Gunderson JG: A BPD Brief: An Introduction to Borderline Personality Disorder Diagnosis, Origins, Course, and Treatment. Washington, NJ, National Education Alliance for Borderline Personality Disorder, 2006

Gunderson JG: Disturbed relationships as a phenotype for borderline personality disorder. Am J Psychiatry 164(11):1637–1640, 2007 17974925

Gunderson JG, Berkowitz C: Family Guidelines: Multiple Family Group Program at McLean Hospital. Belmont, MA, New England Personality Disorder Association, 2006

Gunderson JG, Links PS: Borderline Personality Disorder: A Clinical Guide, Second Edition. Washington, DC, American Psychiatric Association Publishing, 2008

Gunderson JG, Links P: Handbook of Good Psychiatric Management for Borderline Personality Disorder. Washington, DC, American Psychiatric Publishing, 2014, p 180

Gunderson JG, Lyons-Ruth K: BPD's interpersonal hypersensitivity phenotype: a gene-environment-developmental model. J Pers Disord 22(1):22–41, 2008 18312121

Gunderson JG, Shea MT, Skodol AE, et al: The Collaborative Longitudinal Personality Disorders Study: development, aims, design, and sample characteristics. J Pers Disord 14(4):300–315, 2000 11213788

Gunderson JG, Bender D, Sanislow C, et al: Plausibility and possible determinants of sudden "remissions" in borderline patients. Psychiatry 66(2):111–119, 2003 12868289

Gunderson JG, Morey LC, Stout RL, et al: Major depressive disorder and borderline personality disorder revisited: longitudinal interactions. J Clin Psychiatry 65(8):1049–1056, 2004

Gunderson JG, Weinberg I, Daversa MT, et al: Descriptive and longitudinal observations on the relationship of borderline personality disorder and bipolar disorder. Am J Psychiatry 163(7):1173–1178, 2006 16816221

Gunderson JG, Stout RL, McGlashan TH, et al: Ten-year course of borderline personality disorder: psychopathology and function from the Collaborative Longitudinal Personality Disorders study. Arch Gen Psychiatry 68(8):827–837, 2011 21464343

Gunderson JG, Herpertz SC, Skodol AE, et al: Borderline personality disorder. Nat Rev Dis Primers 4:18029, 2018 29795363

Gutheil TG: Suicide, suicide litigation, and borderline personality disorder. J Pers Disord 18(3):248–256, 2004 15237045

Hamann J, Bühner M, Rüsch N: Self-stigma and consumer participation in shared decision making in mental health services. Psychiatr Serv 68(8):783–788, 2017 28412895

Hamza CA, Stewart SL, Willoughby T: Examining the link between nonsuicidal self-injury and suicidal behavior: a review of the literature and an integrated model. Clin Psychol Rev 32(6):482–495, 2012 22717336

Hanegraaf L, van Baal S, Hohwy J, Verdejo-Garcia A: A systematic review and meta-analysis of "Systems for Social Processes" in borderline personality and substance use disorders. Neurosci Biobehav Rev 127:572–592, 2021 33865874

Harrison TF, Connery HS: The Complete Family Guide to Addiction: Everything You Need to Know Now to Help Your Loved One and Yourself. New York, Guilford Press, 2019

Harned MS, Chapman AL, Dexter-Mazza ET, et al: Treating co-occurring Axis I disorders in recurrently suicidal women with borderline personality disorder: a 2-year randomized trial of dialectical behavior therapy versus community treatment by experts. J Consult Clin Psychol 76(6):1068–1075, 2008 19045974

Hasin DS, Wall M, Witkiewitz K, et al; Alcohol Clinical Trials Initiative (AC-TIVE) Workgroup: Change in non-abstinent WHO drinking risk levels and alcohol dependence: a 3 year follow-up study in the US general population. Lancet Psychiatry 4(6):469–476, 2017 28456501

Heinälä P, Alho H, Kiianmaa K, et al: Targeted use of naltrexone without prior detoxification in the treatment of alcohol dependence: a factorial double-blind, placebo-controlled trial. J Clin Psychopharmacol 21(3):287–292, 2001 11386491

Hendler RA, Ramchandani VA, Gilman J, Hommer DW: Stimulant and sedative effects of alcohol, in Behavioral Neurobiology of Alcohol Addiction, Vol. 13. Edited by Sommer EWH, Spanagel R. Berlin, Springer, 2011, pp 489–509

Hepp J, Kieslich PJ, Schmitz M, et al: Negativity on two sides: individuals with borderline personality disorder form negative first impressions of others and are perceived negatively by them. Personal Disord 12(6):514–525, 2021 32881574

Hermens ML, van Splunteren PT, van den Bosch A, Verheul R: Barriers to implementing the clinical guideline on borderline personality disorder in the Netherlands. Psychiatr Serv 62(11):1381–1383, 2011 22211222

Hill KP, Gold MS, Nemeroff CB, et al: Risks and benefits of cannabis and cannabinoids in psychiatry. Am J Psychiatry 179(2):98–109, 2022 34875873

Hoffman NG: ASAM Patient Placement Criteria for the Treatment of Psychoactive Substance Use Disorders. Rockville, MD, American Society of Addiction Medicine, 1993

Hong V: Borderline personality disorder in the emergency department: good psychiatric management. Harv Rev Psychiatry 24(5):357–366, 2016 27603743

Hong V: Emergency departments, in Applications of Good Psychiatric Management for Borderline Personality Disorder. Edited by Choi-Kain LW, Gunderson JG. Washington, DC, American Psychiatric Association Publishing, 2019, pp 37–56

Howard KP, Cheavens JS: Interpersonal emotion regulation in the context of social networks: a focus on borderline personality disorder. Personal Disord 14(2):182–185, 2023 35446102

Hudon A, Gaudreau-Ménard C, Bouchard-Boivin M, et al: The use of computer-driven technologies in the treatment of borderline personality disorder: a systematic review. J Clin Med 11(13):3685, 2022 35806970

Iliakis EA, Sonley AKI, Ilagan GS, Choi-Kain LW: Treatment of borderline personality disorder: is supply adequate to meet public health needs? Psychiatr Serv 70(9):772–781, 2019 31138059

Iliakis EA, Ilagan GS, Choi-Kain LW: Dropout rates from psychotherapy trials for borderline personality disorder: a meta-analysis. Personal Disord 12(3):193–206, 2021

Ingkachotivanich N, Wongpakaran T, Wongpakaran N, et al: Different effects of perceived social support on the relationship between perceived stress and depression among university students with borderline personality disorder symptoms: a multigroup mediation analysis. Healthcare (Basel) 10(11):2212, 2022

Isaacs JY, Smith MM, Sherry SB, et al: Alcohol use and death by suicide: a meta-analysis of 33 studies. Suicide Life Threat Behav 52(4):600–614, 2022 35181905

Iskric A, Barkley-Levenson E: Neural changes in borderline personality disorder after dialectical behavior therapy-a review. Front Psychiatry 12:772081, 2021 34975574

Iyahen EO, Omoruyi OO, Rowa-Dewar N, Dobbie F: Exploring the barriers and facilitators to the uptake of smoking cessation services for people in treatment or recovery from problematic drug or alcohol use: a qualitative systematic review. PLoS One 18(7):e0288409, 2023 37440505

Jacob KL: Clinical observations about the potential benefits and pitfalls of between-session contacts with borderline patients. Harv Rev Psychiatr 24(5):e8–e14, 2016

Jahng S, Solhan MB, Tomko RL, et al: Affect and alcohol use: an ecological momentary assessment study of outpatients with borderline personality disorder. J Abnorm Psychol 120(3):572–584, 2011 21823761

Johns Hopkins Medicine. CAGE Substance Abuse Screening Tool. Baltimore, Johns Hopkins School of Medicine, n.d. Available at: https://www.hopkins-

medicine.org/-/media/johns-hopkins-health-plans/documents/all_plans/
cage-substance-screening-tool.pdf. Accessed March 4, 2024.

Johnson BA, Ait-Daoud N, Bowden CL, et al: Oral topiramate for treatment of
alcohol dependence: a randomised controlled trial. Lancet 361(9370):1677–
1685, 2003 12767733

Johnson BA, Ait-Daoud N, Akhtar FZ, Ma JZ: Oral topiramate reduces the consequences of drinking and improves the quality of life of alcohol-dependent
individuals: a randomized controlled trial. Arch Gen Psychiatry 61(9):905–
912, 2004 15351769

Johnson BA, Rosenthal N, Capece JA, et al; Topiramate for Alcoholism Advisory
Board; Topiramate for Alcoholism Study Group: Topiramate for treating alcohol dependence: a randomized controlled trial. JAMA 298(14):1641–
1651, 2007 17925516

Jonas DE, Amick HR, Feltner C, et al: Pharmacotherapy for adults with alcohol
use disorders in outpatient settings: a systematic review and meta-analysis.
JAMA 311(18):1889–1900, 2014 24825644

Jordan JA: Alcoholics Anonymous: a vehicle for achieving capacity for secure attachment relationships and adaptive affect regulation. J Soc Work Pract Addict 19(3):201–222, 2019

Kapur N, Cooper J, O'Connor RC, Hawton K: Non-suicidal self-injury v. attempted suicide: new diagnosis or false dichotomy? Br J Psychiatry
202(5):326–328, 2013 23637107

Karno MP, Longabaugh R: Less directiveness by therapists improves drinking
outcomes of reactant clients in alcoholism treatment. J Consult Clin Psychol
73(2):262–267, 2005 15796633

Kaskutas LA, Bond J, Humphreys K: Social networks as mediators of the effect
of Alcoholics Anonymous. Addiction 97(7):891–900, 2002 12133128

Kaufman EA, Perez J, Lazarus S, et al: Understanding the association between
borderline personality disorder and alcohol-related problems: an examination of drinking motives, impulsivity, and affective instability. Personal Disord 11(3):213–221, 2020 31724410

Kelly JF: The protective wall of human community: the new evidence on the clinical and public health utility of twelve-step mutual-help organizations and
related treatments. Psychiatr Clin North Am 45(3):557–575, 2022 36055739

Kelly JF, Eddie D: The role of spirituality and religiousness in aiding recovery
from alcohol and other drug problems: an investigation in a national U.S.
sample. Psychol Relig Spiritual 12(1):116–123, 2020 33767804

Kelly JF, Hoeppner BB: Does Alcoholics Anonymous work differently for men
and women? A moderated multiple-mediation analysis in a large clinical
sample. Drug Alcohol Depend 130(1–3):186–193, 2013 23206376

Kelly JF, Stout RL, Magill M, et al: Spirituality in recovery: a lagged mediational
analysis of alcoholics anonymous' principal theoretical mechanism of behavior change. Alcohol (Hanover) 35(3):454–463, 2011 21158876

Kelly JF, Greene MC, Bergman B, et al: The sponsor alliance inventory: assessing the therapeutic bond between 12-step attendees and their sponsors. Alcohol Alcohol 51(1):32–39, 2016a 26113488

Kelly JF, Greene MC, Bergman BG: Recovery benefits of the "therapeutic alliance" among 12-step mutual-help organization attendees and their sponsors. Drug Alcohol Depend 162:64–71, 2016b 26961963

Kelly JF, Bergman B, Hoeppner BB, et al: Prevalence and pathways of recovery from drug and alcohol problems in the United States population: implications for practice, research, and policy. Drug Alcohol Depend 181:162–169, 2017 29055821

Kelly JF, Humphreys K, Ferri M: Alcoholics Anonymous and other 12-step programs for alcohol use disorder. Cochrane Database Syst Rev 3(3):CD012880, 2020 32159228

Kelly JF, Greene MC, Abry A: A US national randomized study to guide how best to reduce stigma when describing drug-related impairment in practice and policy. Addiction 116(7):1757–1767, 2021 33197084

Kendler KS, Myers J, Reichborn-Kjennerud T: Borderline personality disorder traits and their relationship with dimensions of normative personality: a web-based cohort and twin study. Acta Psychiatr Scand 123(5):349–359, 2011 21198457

Keuroghlian AS, Palmer BA, Choi-Kain LW, et al: The effect of attending good psychiatric management (GPM) workshops on attitudes toward patients with borderline personality disorder. J Pers Disord 30(4):567–576, 2016 26111249

Khemiri L, Jokinen J, Runeson B, Jayaram-Lindström N: Suicide risk associated with experience of violence and impulsivity in alcohol dependent patients. Sci Rep 6(1):19373, 2016 26784730

Kienast T, Stoffers J, Bermpohl F, Lieb K: Borderline personality disorder and comorbid addiction: epidemiology and treatment. Dtsch Arztebl Int 111(16):280–286, 2014 24791755

Kilian C, Manthey J, Carr S, et al: Stigmatization of people with alcohol use disorders: an updated systematic review of population studies. Alcohol (Hanover) 45(5):899–911, 2021 33970504

Klein P, Fairweather AK, Lawn S: Structural stigma and its impact on healthcare for borderline personality disorder: a scoping review. Int J Ment Health Syst 16(1):48, 2022 36175958

Kolla NJ, Links PS, McMain S, et al: Demonstrating adherence to guidelines for the treatment of patients with borderline personality disorder. Can J Psychiatry 54(3):181–189, 2009 19321022

Kolly S, Despland JN, de Roten Y, et al: Therapist adherence to good psychiatric practice in a short-term treatment for borderline personality disorder. J Nerv Ment Dis 204(7):489–493, 2016 27187770

Koob GF, Volkow ND: Neurobiology of addiction: a neurocircuitry analysis. Lancet Psychiatry 3(8):760–773, 2016 27475769

Kozak K, Lucatch AM, Lowe DJE, et al: The neurobiology of impulsivity and substance use disorders: implications for treatment. Ann N Y Acad Sci 1451(1):71–91, 2019 30291624

Knight RP: Borderline states. Bull Menninger Clin 17:1–12, 1953

Knipe D, Padmanathan P, Newton-Howes G, et al: Suicide and self-harm. Lancet 399(10338):1903–1916, 2022 35512727

Kramer U: Good psychiatric management: does it have a "good enough" empirical basis? Am J Psychother (in press) 2024

Kramer U, Berger T, Kolly S, et al: Effects of motive-oriented therapeutic relationship in early phase treatment of borderline personality disorder: a pilot study of a randomized trial. J Nerv Ment Dis 199(4):244–250, 2011 21451348

Kramer U, Kolly S, Berthoud L, et al: Effects of motive-oriented therapeutic relationship in a ten-session general psychiatric treatment of borderline personality disorder: a randomized controlled trial. Psychother Psychosom 83(3):176–186, 2014 24752034

Kramer U, Stulz N, Berthoud L, et al: The shorter the better? A follow-up analysis of 10-session psychiatric treatment including the motive-oriented therapeutic relationship for borderline personality disorder. Psychother Res 27(3):362–370, 2017 26684670

Kramer U, Kolly S, Charbon P, et al: Brief psychiatric treatment for borderline personality disorder as a first step of care: adapting general psychiatric management to a 10-session intervention. Person Disord 13(5):516–526, 2022

Kranzler HR: Overview of alcohol use disorder. Am J Psychiatry 180(8):565–572, 2023 37525595

Kranzler HR, Gage A: Acamprosate efficacy in alcohol-dependent patients: summary of results from three pivotal trials. Am J Addict 17(1):70–76, 2008 18214726

Kranzler HR, Armeli S, Tennen H, et al: Targeted naltrexone for early problem drinkers. J Clin Psychopharmacol 23(3):294–304, 2003 12826991

Kranzler HR, Feinn R, Morris P, Hartwell EE: A meta-analysis of the efficacy of gabapentin for treating alcohol use disorder. Addiction 114(9):1547–1555, 2019 31077485

Krebs P, Norcross JC, Nicholson JM, Prochaska JO: Stages of change and psychotherapy outcomes: a review and meta-analysis. J Clin Psychol 74(11):1964–1979, 2018 30335193

Krentzman AR, Robinson EAR, Perron BE, Cranford JA: Predictors of membership in Alcoholics Anonymous in a sample of successfully remitted alcoholics. J Psychoactive Drugs 43(1):20–26, 2011 21615004

Krentzman AR, Strobbe S, Harris JI, et al: Decreased drinking and Alcoholics Anonymous are associated with different dimensions of spirituality. Psychol Relig Spiritual 9(Suppl 1):S40–S48, 2017 29057032

Kuerbis A, Tonigan JS: More than taking a chair: the perceived group social dynamics of alcoholics anonymous related to changes in spiritual practices. Alcohol Treat Q 36(3):314–329, 2018 30397366

Lamis DA, Malone PS: Alcohol-related problems and risk of suicide among college students: the mediating roles of belongingness and burdensomeness. Suicide Life Threat Behav 41(5):543–553, 2011 21883409

Lane SP, Carpenter RW, Sher KJ, Trull TJ: Alcohol craving and consumption in borderline personality disorder: when, where, and with whom. Clin Psychol Sci 4(5):775–792, 2016 28042520

Lange S, Jiang H, Kaplan MS, et al: Association between acute alcohol use and firearm-involved suicide in the United States. JAMA Netw Open 6(3):e235248, 2023 36988957

Laporte L, Paris J, Bergevin T, et al: Clinical outcomes of a stepped care program for borderline personality disorder. Personal Ment Health 12(3):252–264, 2018 29709109

Lazarus SA, Southward MW, Cheavens JS: Do borderline personality disorder features and rejection sensitivity predict social network outcomes over time? Pers Individ Dif 100:62–67, 2016

Lazarus SA, Beardslee J, Pedersen SL, Stepp SD: A within-person analysis of the association between borderline personality disorder and alcohol use in adolescents. J Abnorm Child Psychol 45(6):1157–1167, 2017 27812907

Leichsenring F, Heim N, Leweke F, et al: Borderline personality disorder: a review. JAMA 329(8):670–679, 2023 36853245

Lieb K, Völlm B, Rücker G, et al: Pharmacotherapy for borderline personality disorder: Cochrane systematic review of randomised trials. Br J Psychiatry 196(1):4–12, 2010 20044651

Lieberman MD, Eisenberger NI, Crockett MJ, et al: Putting feelings into words: affect labeling disrupts amygdala activity in response to affective stimuli. Psychol Sci 18(5):421–428, 2007 17576282

Likhitsathian S, Uttawichai K, Booncharoen H, et al: Topiramate treatment for alcoholic outpatients recently receiving residential treatment programs: a 12-week, randomized, placebo-controlled trial. Drug Alcohol Depend 133(2):440–446, 2013 23906999

Linehan MM: Cognitive-Behavioral Treatment of Borderline Personality Disorder. New York, Guilford Press, 1993

Linehan MM, Schmidt H 3rd, Dimeff LA, et al: Dialectical behavior therapy for patients with borderline personality disorder and drug-dependence. Am J Addict 8(4):279–292, 1999 10598211

Links PS, Heslegrave RJ, Mitton JE, et al: Borderline personality disorder and substance abuse: consequences of comorbidity. Can J Psychiatry 40(1):9–14, 1995 7874683

Links PS, Gould B, Ratnayake R: Assessing suicidal youth with antisocial, borderline, or narcissistic personality disorder. Can J Psychiatry 48(5):301–310, 2003 12866335

Links P, Ross J: Good psychiatric management of borderline personality disorder: foundations and future challenges. Am J Psychother (in press) 2024

Linnoila MI: Benzodiazepines and alcohol. J Psychiatr Res 24(Suppl 2):121–127, 1990 1980691

Litt MD, Kadden RM, Kabela-Cormier E, Petry NM: Changing network support for drinking: network support project 2-year follow-up. J Consult Clin Psychol 77(2):229–242, 2009 19309183

Lohanan T, Leesawat T, Wongpakaran T, et al: Screening instrument for borderline personality disorder. APA PsychNet, 2020. Available at: https://doi.org/10.1037/t78424-000. Accessed July 3, 2024.

Luoma JB, Chwyl C, Kaplan J: Substance use and shame: a systematic and meta-analytic review. Clin Psychol Rev 70:1–12, 2019 30856404

Luyten P, Blatt SJ: Interpersonal relatedness and self-definition in normal and disrupted personality development: retrospect and prospect. Am Psychol 68(3):172–183, 2013 23586492

Lynch TR, Rosenthal MZ, Kosson DS, et al: Heightened sensitivity to facial expressions of emotion in borderline personality disorder. Emotion 6(4):647–655, 2006 17144755

MacKillop J, Agabio R, Feldstein Ewing SW, et al: Hazardous drinking and alcohol use disorders. Nat Rev Dis Primers 8(1):80, 2022 36550121

Magill M, Kiluk BD, Mccrady BS, et al: Active ingredients of treatment and client mechanisms of change in behavioral treatments for alcohol use disorders: progress 10 years later. Alcohol Clin Exp Res 39(10):1852–1862, 2015

Manning V, Best D, Faulkner N, et al: Does active referral by a doctor or 12-Step peer improve 12-Step meeting attendance? Results from a pilot randomised control trial. Drug Alcohol Depend 126(1–2):131–137, 2012 22677458

Mariani JJ, Pavlicova M, Basaraba C, et al: Pilot randomized placebo-controlled clinical trial of high-dose gabapentin for alcohol use disorder. Alcohol (Hanover) 45(8):1639–1652, 2021 34120336

Martín-Blanco A, Patrizi B, Soler J, et al: Use of nalmefene in patients with comorbid borderline personality disorder and alcohol use disorder: a preliminary report. Int Clin Psychopharmacol 32(4):231–234, 2017 28181957

Masland SR, Price D, MacDonald J, et al: Enduring effects of one-day training in good psychiatric management on clinician attitudes about borderline personality disorder. J Nerv Ment Dis 206(11):865–869, 2018 30371640

Mason BJ, Quello S, Goodell V, et al: Gabapentin treatment for alcohol dependence: a randomized clinical trial. JAMA Intern Med 174(1):70–77, 2014 24190578

Mason BJ, Quello S, Shadan F: Gabapentin for the treatment of alcohol use disorder. Expert Opin Invest Drugs 27(1):113–124, 2018

McGirr A, Paris J, Lesage A, et al: Risk factors for suicide completion in border-line personality disorder: a case-control study of cluster B comorbidity and impulsive aggression. J Clin Psychiatry 68(5):721–729, 2007 17503981

McGlashan TH: Omnipotence, helplessness, and control with the borderline patient. Am J Psychother 37(1):49–61, 1983 6846667

McLellan AT, Kushner H, Metzger D, et al: The fifth edition of the Addiction Severity Index. J Subst Abuse Treat 9(3):199–213, 1992 1334156

McMain SF, Links PS, Gnam WH, et al: A randomized trial of dialectical behavior therapy versus general psychiatric management for borderline personality disorder. Am J Psychiatry 166(12):1365–1374, 2009 19755574

McMain SF, Guimond T, Streiner DL, et al: Dialectical behavior therapy compared with general psychiatric management for borderline personality disorder: clinical outcomes and functioning over a 2-year follow-up. Am J Psychiatry 169(6):650–661, 2012 22581157

Mee-Lee D, Shulman GD: The ASAM placement criteria and matching patients to treatment, in Principles of Addiction Medicine, 3rd Edition. Edited by Graham AW, Schultz TK, Mayo-Smith MF, et al. Chevy Chase, MD, American Society of Addiction Medicine, 2003, pp 453–465

Melson AJ, O'Connor RC: Differentiating adults who think about self-harm from those who engage in self-harm: the role of volitional alcohol factors. BMC Psychiatry 19(1):319, 2019 31660913

Menon NK, Shanafelt TD, Sinsky CA, et al: Association of physician burnout with suicidal ideation and medical errors. JAMA Netw Open 3(12):e2028780, 2020 33295977

Mercer D, Douglass AB, Links PS: Meta-analysis of mood stabilizers, antidepressants and antipsychotics in the treatment of borderline personality disorder: effectiveness for depression and anger symptoms. J Pers Disord 23:156–174, 2009

Meyers RJ, Wolfe BL: Get Your Loved One Sober: Alternatives to Nagging, Pleading, and Threatening. Center City, Minnesota, Hazelden, 2009

Meyers RJ, Miller WR, Smith JE, Tonigan JS: A randomized trial of two methods for engaging treatment-refusing drug users through concerned significant others. J Consult Clin Psychol 70(5):1182–1185, 2002 12362968

Miller FT, Abrams T, Dulit R, Fyer M: Substance abuse in borderline personalityt disorder. Am J Drug Alcohol Abuse 19(4):491–497, 1993

Miller PG: Safe using messages may not be enough to promote behaviour change amongst injecting drug users who are ambivalent or indifferent towards death. Harm Reduct J 6(1):18, 2009 19630988

Miller WR: Motivational interviewing with problem drinkers. Behav Psychother 11(2):147–172, 1983

Miller WR, Rollnick S: Motivational Interviewing: Helping People Change, 4th Edition. New York, Guilford Press, 2023

Miller WR, Meyers RJ, Tonigan JS: Engaging the unmotivated in treatment for alcohol problems: a comparison of three strategies for intervention through family members. J Consult Clin Psychol 67(5):688–697, 1999 10535235

Min J, Mullins-Sweatt S, Widiger TA: Informant five-factor borderline inventory. APA PsychNet, 2021. Available at: https://doi.org/10.1037/t81072-000. Accessed July 3, 2024.

Mirijello A, Sestito L, Antonelli M, et al: Identification and management of acute alcohol intoxication. Eur J Intern Med 108:1–8, 2023 35985955

Modesto-Lowe V, Brooks D, Ghani M: Alcohol dependence and suicidal behavior: from research to clinical challenges. Harv Rev Psychiatry 14(5):241–248, 2006 16990169

Modesto-Lowe V, Barron GC, Aronow B, Chaplin M: Gabapentin for alcohol use disorder: a good option, or cause for concern? Cleveland Clin J Med 86(12):815–823, 2019

Moles A, Kieffer BL, D'Amato FR: Deficit in attachment behavior in mice lacking the mu-opioid receptor gene. Science 304(5679):1983–1986, 2004 15218152

Morana HC, Câmara FP: International guidelines for the management of personality disorders. Curr Opin Psychiatry 19(5):539–543, 2006 16874131

Moreira-Almeida A, Sharma A, van Rensburg BJ, et al: WPA Position Statement on spirituality and religion in psychiatry. World Psychiatry 15(1):87–88, 2016 26833620

Morey LC, Boggs C: The personality assessment inventory (PAI). New York, Wiley and Sons, 2004, pp 15–29

Morgenstern J, Langenbucher J, Labouvie E, Miller KJ: The comorbidity of alcoholism and personality disorders in a clinical population: prevalence rates and relation to alcohol typology variables. J Abnorm Psychol 106(1):74–84, 1997 9103719

Motivational Interviewing Network of Trainers. Available at: www.motivationalinterviewing.org. Accessed March 4, 2024.

Mowbray O, Quinn A, Cranford JA: Social networks and alcohol use disorders: findings from a nationally representative sample. Am J Drug Alcohol Abuse 40(3):181–186, 2014 24405256

Mullins-Sweatt SN, Edmundson M, Sauer-Zavala S, et al: Five-factor measure of borderline personality traits. J Pers Assess 94(5):475–487, 2012

Mutschler J, Grosshans M, Koopmann A, et al: Supervised disulfiram in relapse prevention in alcohol-dependent patients suffering from comorbid borderline personality disorder—a case series. Alcohol Alcohol 45(2):146–150, 2010 20107104

Myrick H, Anton R, Voronin K, et al: A double-blind evaluation of gabapentin on alcohol effects and drinking in a clinical laboratory paradigm. Alcohol Clin Exp Res 31(2):221–227, 2007 17250613

National Institute on Drug Abuse. Instruments. Available at: https://cde.nida.nih.gov/instruments. Accessed March 4, 2024.

Nickel MK, Nickel C, Mitterlehner FO, et al: Topiramate treatment of aggression in female borderline personality disorder patients: a double-blind, placebo-controlled study. J Clin Psychiatry 65(11):1515–1519, 2004

Nickel MK, Nickel C, Kaplan P, et al: Treatment of aggression with topiramate in male borderline patients: a double-blind, placebo-controlled study. Biol Psychiatry 57(5):495–499, 2005 15737664

Nock MK, Prinstein MJ: A functional approach to the assessment of self-mutilative behavior. J Consult Clin Psychol 72(5):885–890, 2004 15482046

NovoPsych: McLean Screening Instrument for BPD (MSI-BPD). Melbourne, Australia, NovoPsych, n.d. Available at: https://novopsych.com.au/wp-content/uploads/2023/02/msi-bpd-borderline-personality-disorder-assessment-blank-form.pdf. Accessed July 3, 2024

Nowinski J, Baker S: The Twelve-Step Facilitation Handbook: A Systematic Approach to Early Recovery From Alcoholism and Addiction. Hoboken, NJ, Jossey-Bass, 1992

O'Farrell TJ, Fals-Stewart W: Behavioral couples and family therapy for substance abusers. Curr Psychiatry Rep 4(5):371–376, 2002

O'Malley SS, Jaffe AJ, Chang G, et al: Six-month follow-up of naltrexone and psychotherapy for alcohol dependence. Arch Gen Psychiatry 53(3):217–224, 1996 8611058

Oud M, Arntz A, Hermens ML, et al: Specialized psychotherapies for adults with borderline personality disorder: a systematic review and meta-analysis. Aust N Z J Psychiatry 52(10):949–961, 2018 30091375

Packman WL, O'Connor Pennuto T, Bongar B, Orthwein J: Legal issues of professional negligence in suicide cases. Behav Sci Law 22(5):697–713, 2004

Pagano ME, White WL, Kelly JF, et al: The 10-year course of Alcoholics Anonymous participation and long-term outcomes: a follow-up study of outpatient subjects in Project MATCH. Subst Abus 34(1):51–59, 2013 23327504

Paris J: Chronic suicidality among patients with borderline personality disorder. Psychiatr Serv 53(6):738–742, 2002 12045312

Paris J: Is hospitalization useful for suicidal patients with borderline personality disorder? J Pers Disord 18(3):240–247, 2004

Paris J: Stepped care: an alternative to routine extended treatment for patients with borderline personality disorder. Psychiatr Serv 64(10):1035–1037, 2013 23945913

Paris J, Zweig-Frank H: A 27-year follow-up of patients with borderline personality disorder. Compr Psychiatry 42(6):482–487, 2001 11704940

Pennay A, Cameron J, Reichert T, et al: A systematic review of interventions for co-occurring substance use disorder and borderline personality disorder. J Subst Abuse Treat 41(4):363–373, 2011 21742460

Penzenstadler L, Kolly S, Rothen S, et al: Effects of substance use disorder on treatment process and outcome in a ten-session psychiatric treatment for borderline personality disorder. Subst Abuse Treat Prev Policy 13(1):10, 2018 29482597

Perez J, Beale E, Overholser J, et al: Depression and alcohol use disorders as precursors to death by suicide. Death Stud 46(3):619–627, 2022 32238058

Peris L, Szerman N, Ruíz M: Efficacy and safety of gabapentin in borderline personality disorder: a six-month, open-label study [in Spanish]. Vertex 18(76):418–422, 2007 18273430

Pfund RA, Hallgren KA, Maisto SA, et al: Dose of psychotherapy and long-term recovery outcomes: an examination of attendance patterns in alcohol use disorder treatment. J Consult Clin Psychol 89(12):1026–1034, 2021 35025543

Piccinelli M, Tessari E, Bortolomasi M, et al: Efficacy of the alcohol use disorders identification test as a screening tool for hazardous alcohol intake and related disorders in primary care: a validity study. BMJ 314(7078):420–424, 1997 9040389

Pilar MR, Eyler AA, Moreland-Russell S, Brownson RC: Actual causes of death in relation to media, policy, and funding attention: examining public health priorities. Front Public Health 8:279, 2020 32733836

Price D: Generalist adult outpatient psychiatry practice, in Applications of Good Psychiatric Management for Borderline Personality Disorder. Edited by Choi-Kain LW, Gunderson JG. Washington, DC, American Psychiatric Association Publishing, 2019, pp 85–116

Prochaska JO, DiClemente CC: Transtheoretical therapy: toward a more integrative model of change. Psychotherapy (Chic) 19(3):276–288, 1982

Quaytman M, Sharfstein SS: Treatment for borderline personality disorder in 1987 and 1997. Am J Psychiatr 154(8):1139–1144, 1997

Ralevski E, Ball S, Nich C, et al: The impact of personality disorders on alcohol-use outcomes in a pharmacotherapy trial for alcohol dependence and comorbid Axis I disorders. Am J Addict 16(6):443–449, 2007 18058408

Rehm J: The risks associated with alcohol use and alcoholism. Alcohol Res Health 34(2):135–143, 2011

Rehm J, Dawson D, Frick U, et al: Burden of disease associated with alcohol use disorders in the United States. Alcohol (Hanover) 38(4):1068–1077, 2014 24428196

Reichl C, Kaess M: Self-harm in the context of borderline personality disorder. Curr Opin Psychol 37:139–144, 2021 33548678

Rentsch CT, Fiellin DA, Bryant KJ, et al: Association between gabapentin receipt for any indication and alcohol use disorders identification test-consumption scores among clinical subpopulations with and without alcohol use disorder. Alcohol (Hanover) 43(3):522–530, 2019 30620410

Rentsch CT, Morford KL, Fiellin DA, et al: Safety of gabapentin prescribed for any indication in a large clinical cohort of 571,718 US veterans with and without alcohol use disorder. Alcohol (Hanover) 44(9):1807–1815, 2020 32628784

Richman Czégel MJ, Unoka Z, Dudas RB, Demetrovics Z: Rumination in borderline personality disorder: a meta-analytic review. J Pers Disord 36(4):399–412, 2022 35913769

Ridolfi ME, Rossi R, Occhialini G, Gunderson JG: A clinical trial of a psychoeducation group intervention for patients with borderline personality disorder. J Clin Psychiatry 81(1):19m12753, 2019

Rigotti NA, Kruse GR, Livingstone-Banks J, Hartmann-Boyce J: Treatment of tobacco smoking: a review. JAMA 327(6):566–577, 2022 35133411

Roozen HG, de Waart R, van der Kroft P: Community reinforcement and family training: an effective option to engage treatment-resistant substance-abusing individuals in treatment. Addiction 1729–1738, 2010

Roth AS, Ostroff RB, Hoffman RE: Naltrexone as a treatment for repetitive self-injurious behaviour: an open-label trial. J Clin Psychiatry 57(6):233–237, 1996

Ruocco AC, Carcone D: A neurobiological model of borderline personality disorder: systematic and integrative review. Harv Rev Psychiatry 24(5):311–329, 2016 27603741

Ryan EP, Oquendo MA: Suicide risk assessment and prevention: challenges and opportunities. Focus Am Psychiatr Publ 18(2):88–99, 2020 33162846

Ryle A, Golynkina K: Effectiveness of time-limited cognitive analytic therapy of borderline personality disorder: factors associated with outcome. Br J Med Psychol 73(Pt2):197–210, 2000

Sakinofsky I: The aftermath of suicide: managing survivors' bereavement. Can J Psychiatry 52(6)(Suppl 1):129S–136S, 2007 17824358

Sansone RA, Kelley AR, Forbis JS: Religion/spirituality status and borderline personality symptomatology among outpatients in an internal medicine clinic. Int J Psychiatry Clin Pract 16(1):48–52, 2012 22122648

Schulze L, Schmahl C, Niedtfeld I: Neural correlates of disturbed emotion processing in borderline personality disorder: a multimodal meta-analysis. Biol Psychiatry 79(2):97–106, 2016 25935068

Schuppert HM, Timmerman ME, Bloo J, et al: Emotion regulation training for adolescents with borderline personality disorder traits: a randomized controlled trial. J Am Acad Child Adolesc Psychiatry 51(12):1314–1323.e2, 2012 23200288

Schweizer E, Rickels K, De Martinis N, et al: The effect of personality on withdrawal severity and taper outcome in benzodiazepine dependent patients. Psychol Med 28(3):713–720, 1998

Scribd: Borderline Symptom List 23. San Francisco, Scribd, n.d. Available at: https://www.scribd.com/document/373087907/Borderline-Personality-Disorder-Scale-pdf. Accessed July 3, 2024

Segher K, Huys L, Desmet T, et al: Recognition of a disulfiram ethanol reaction in the emergency department is not always straightforward. PLoS One 15(12):e0243222, 2020 33270785

Shanks C, Pfohl B, Blum N, Black DW: Can negative attitudes toward patients with borderline personality disorder be changed? The effect of attending a STEPPS workshop. J Pers Disord 25(6):806–812, 2011 22217226

Shapiro-Thompson R, Fineberg SK: The state of overmedication in borderline personality disorder: interpersonal and structural factors. Curr Treat Options Psychiatry 9(1):1–13, 2022 36185615

Sharp C: Personality disorders. N Engl J Med 387(10):916–923, 2022 36069872

Sharp C, Wall K: Personality pathology grows up: adolescence as a sensitive period. Curr Opin Psychol 21:111–116, 2018 29227834

Sharp C, Wright AGC, Fowler JC, et al: The structure of personality pathology: both general ('g') and specific ('s') factors? J Abnorm Psychol 124(2):387–398, 2015 25730515

Silk KR, Faurino L: Psychopharmacology of personality disorders, in The Oxford Handbook of Personality Disorders. Edited by Widiger T. London, Oxford University Press, 2012, pp 712–726

Sinclair J, O'Neill A: Update on the management of alcohol use disorders. BJPsych Adv 26(2):82–91, 2020

Skoglund C, Tiger A, Rück C, et al: Familial risk and heritability of diagnosed borderline personality disorder: a register study of the Swedish population. Mol Psychiatry 26(3):999–1008, 2021 31160693

Smith JE, Myers RJ: The CRAFT Treatment Manual for Substance Use Problems: Working With Family Members. New York, Guilford Press, 2023

Soni A, Thiyagarajan A, Reeve J: Feasibility and effectiveness of deprescribing benzodiazepines and Z-drugs: systematic review and meta-analysis. Addiction 118(1):7–16, 2023 35815384

Sonley AK, Choi-Kain LW (eds): Good Psychiatric Management and Dialectical Behavioral Therapy: A Clinician's Guide to Integration and Stepped Care. Washington, DC, American Psychiatric Association Publishing, 2021

Sonne S, Rubey R, Brady K, et al: Naltrexone treatment of self-injurious thoughts and behaviors. J Nerv Ment Dis 184(3):192–195, 1996 8600226

Spear LP: Effects of adolescent alcohol consumption on the brain and behaviour. Nat Rev Neurosci 19(4):197–214, 2018 29467469

Srisurapanont M, Jarusuraisin N: Naltrexone for the treatment of alcoholism: a meta-analysis of randomized controlled trials. Int J Neuropsychopharmacol 8(2):267–280, 2005 15850502

Stanley B, Brown GK: Safety planning intervention: a brief intervention to mitigate suicide risk. Cogn Behav Pract 19(2):256–264, 2012

Stavro K, Pelletier J, Potvin S: Widespread and sustained cognitive deficits in alcoholism: a meta-analysis. Addict Biol 18(2):203–213, 2013 22264351

Stepp SD, Trull TJ, Sher KJ: Borderline personality features predict alcohol use problems. J Pers Disord 19(6):711–722, 2005 16553564

Stout RL, Kelly JF, Magill M, Pagano ME: Association between social influences and drinking outcomes across three years. J Stud Alcohol Drugs 73(3):489–497, 2012 22456254

Subbaraman MS, Kaskutas LA, Zemore S: Sponsorship and service as mediators of the effects of Making Alcoholics Anonymous Easier (MAAEZ), a 12-step facilitation intervention. Drug Alcohol Depend 116(1–3):117–124, 2011 21288660

Substance Abuse and Mental Health Services Administration: Substance Abuse: Clinical Issues in Intensive Outpatient Treatment. A Treatment Improvement Protocol. TIP 47. SAMHSA, 2006. Available at: https://store.samhsa. gov/product/tip-47-substance-abuse-clinical-issues-intensive-outpatient-treatment/sma13-4182. Accessed March 25, 2024.

Substance Abuse and Mental Health Services Administration: Key Substance Use and Mental Health Indicators in the United States: Results From the 2020 National Survey on Drug Use and Health. HHS Publ. No. PEP21-07-01-003, NSDUH Series H-56). Rockville, MD, Center for Behavioral Health Statistics and Quality, Substance Abuse and Mental Health Services Administration, 2021a. Available at: https://www.samhsa.gov/data/sites/default/files/reports/rpt35325/NSDUHFFRPDFWHTMLFiles2020/2020 NSDUHFFR1PDFW102121.pdf. Accessed February 20, 2024.

Sullivan JT, Sykora K, Schneiderman J, et al: Assessment of alcohol withdrawal: the revised clinical institute withdrawal assessment for alcohol scale (CIWA-Ar). Br J Addict 84(11):1353–1357, 1989 2597811

Swannell SV, Martin GE, Page A, et al: Prevalence of nonsuicidal self-injury in nonclinical samples: systematic review, meta-analysis and meta-regression. Suicide Life Threat Behav 44(3):273–303, 2014

Sweeney MM, Holtyn AF, Stitzer ML, Gastfriend DR: Practical technology for expanding and improving substance use disorder treatment: telehealth, remote monitoring, and digital health interventions. Psychiatr Clin North Am 45(3):515–528, 2022 36055736

Tate AE, Sahlin H, Liu S, et al: Borderline personality disorder: associations with psychiatric disorders, somatic illnesses, trauma, and adverse behaviors. Mol Psychiatry 27(5):2514–2521, 2022 35304564

Temes CM, Frankenburg FR, Fitzmaurice GM, Zanarini MC: Deaths by suicide and other causes among patients with borderline personality disorder and personality-disordered comparison subjects over 24 years of prospective follow-up. J Clin Psychiatry 80(1):18m12436, 2019 30688417

Thadani B, Pérez-García AM, Bermúdez J: Functional impairment in borderline personality disorder: the mediating role of perceived social support. Front Psychol 13:883833, 2022 35712170

Thompson RG Jr, Eaton NR, Hu M-C, Hasin DS: Borderline personality disorder and regularly drinking alcohol before sex. Drug Alcohol Rev 36(4):540–545, 2017 28321919

Tomko RL, Trull TJ, Wood PK, Sher KJ: Characteristics of borderline personality disorder in a community sample: comorbidity, treatment utilization, and general functioning. J Pers Disord 28(5):734–750, 2014 25248122

Tonigan JS, Rice SL: Is it beneficial to have an Alcoholics Anonymous sponsor? Psychol Addict Behav 24(3):397–403, 2010 20853924

Tonigan JS, Rynes KN, McCrady BS: Spirituality as a change mechanism in 12-step programs: a replication, extension, and refinement. Subst Use Misuse 48(12):1161–1173, 2013 24041178

Tonigan JS, McCallion EA, Frohe T, Pearson MR: Lifetime Alcoholics Anonymous attendance as a predictor of spiritual gains in the Relapse Replication and Extension Project (RREP). Psychol Addict Behav 31(1):54–60, 2017 28080094

Torgersen S, Lygren S, Oien PA, et al: A twin study of personality disorders. Compr Psychiatry 41(6):416–425, 2000 11086146

Trivedi MH, Walker R, Ling W, et al: Bupropion and naltrexone in methamphetamine use disorder. N Engl J Med 384(2):140–153, 2021 33497547

Trull TJ, Sher KJ, Minks-Brown C, et al: Borderline personality disorder and substance use disorders: a review and integration. Clin Psychol Rev 20(2):235–253, 2000 10721499

Trull TJ, Jahng S, Tomko RL, et al: Revised NESARC personality disorder diagnoses: gender, prevalence, and comorbidity with substance dependence disorders. J Pers Disord 24(4):412–426, 2010 20695803

Trull TJ, Freeman LK, Vebares TJ, et al: Borderline personality disorder and substance use disorders: an updated review. Borderline Personal Disord Emot Dysregul 5:15, 2018 30250740

University of Washington: Borderline personality disorder and substance use disorders: an updated review. Seattle, University of Washington, n.d. Available at: https://depts.washington.edu/uwbrtc/wp-content/uploads/Borderline-Symptom-List-BLS-23.pdf. Accessed July 3, 2024

van den Bosch LM, Verheul R, Schippers GM, van den Brink W: Dialectical behavior therapy of borderline patients with and without substance use problems: implementation and long-term effects. Addict Behav 27(6):911–923, 2002 12369475

Van Orden KA, Witte TK, Cukrowicz KC, et al: The interpersonal theory of suicide. Psychol Rev 117(2):575–600, 2010 20438238

Vasilaki EI, Hosier SG, Cox WM: The efficacy of motivational interviewing as a brief intervention for excessive drinking: a meta-analytic review. Alcohol Alcohol 41(3):328–335, 2006 16547122

Vederhus JK, Timko C, Kristensen O, et al: Motivational intervention to enhance post-detoxification 12-Step group affiliation: a randomized controlled trial. Addiction 109(5):766–773, 2014 24400937

Verhulst B, Neale MC, Kendler KS: The heritability of alcohol use disorders: a meta-analysis of twin and adoption studies. Psychol Med 45(5):1061–1072, 2015 25171596

Videler AC, Hutsebaut J, Schulkens JEM, et al: A life span perspective on borderline personality disorder. Curr Psychiatry Rep 21(7):51, 2019 31161404

Vijay NR, Links PS: New frontiers in the role of hospitalization for patients with personality disorders. Curr Psychiatry Rep 9(1):63–67, 2007 17257516

Vungkhanching M, Sher KJ, Jackson KM, Parra GR: Relation of attachment style to family history of alcoholism and alcohol use disorders in early adulthood. Drug Alcohol Depend 75(1):47–53, 2004 15225888

Walter M, Gunderson JG, Zanarini MC, et al: New onsets of substance use disorders in borderline personality disorder over 7 years of follow-ups: findings from the Collaborative Longitudinal Personality Disorders Study. Addiction 104(1):97–103, 2009 19133893

Wiebe RP, Griffin AM, Zheng Y, et al: Twelve steps, two factors: coping strategies moderate the association between craving and daily 12-step use in a college recovery community. Subst Use Misuse 53(1):114–127, 2018 28813187

Wilcox HC, Conner KR, Caine ED: Association of alcohol and drug use disorders and completed suicide: an empirical review of cohort studies. Drug Alcohol Depend 76(Suppl):S11–S19, 2004

Wilson ST, Fertuck EA, Kwitel A, et al: Impulsivity, suicidality and alcohol use disorders in adolescents and young adults with borderline personality disorder. Int J Adolesc Med Health 18(1):189–196, 2006 16639873

Winnicott DW: Transitional objects and transitional phenomena: a study of the first not-me possession. Int J Psychoanal 34(2):89–97, 1953 13061115

Witbrodt J, Kaskutas LA: Does diagnosis matter? Differential effects of 12-step participation and social networks on abstinence. Am J Drug Alcohol Abuse 31(4):685–707, 2005 16320441

Witbrodt J, Kaskutas L, Bond J, Delucchi K: Does sponsorship improve outcomes above Alcoholics Anonymous attendance? A latent class growth curve analysis. Addiction 107(2):301–311, 2012 21752145

Witbrodt J, Ye Y, Bond J, et al: Alcohol and drug treatment involvement, 12-step attendance and abstinence: 9-year cross-lagged analysis of adults in an integrated health plan. J Subst Abuse Treat 46(4):412–419, 2014 24342024

Wnuk M: Religious–spiritual sources of hope and the meaning of life in alcohol co-dependent subjects receiving support in self-help groups. J Subst Use 20(3):194–199, 2015

Wnuk M: Hope as an important factor for mental health in alcohol-dependent subjects attending Alcoholics Anonymous. J Subst Use 22(2):182–186, 2017

Wnuk M: Indirect relationship between Alcoholics Anonymous spirituality and their hopelessness: the role of meaning in life, hope, and abstinence duration. Religions (Basel) 12(11):934, 2021

Wnuk M: The beneficial role of involvement in Alcoholics Anonymous for existential and subjective well-being of alcohol-dependent individuals? The model verification. Int J Environ Res Public Health 19(9):5173, 2022 35564567

Wnuk S, McMain S, Links PS, et al: Factors related to dropout from treatment in two outpatient treatments for borderline personality disorder. J Pers Disord 27(6):716–726, 2013 23718760

World Health Organization: Global Status Report on Alcohol and Health. WHO, 2014. Available at: https://www.who.int/publications-detail-redirect/global-status-report-on-alcohol-and-health-2014. Accessed February 20, 2024.

World Health Organization: International Classification of Diseases, 11th Revision. Geneva, WHO, 2022

Wright AG, Hopwood CJ, Skodol AE, Morey LC: Longitudinal validation of general and specific structural features of personality pathology. J Abnorm Psychol 125(8):1120–1134, 2016a 27819472

Wright AGC, Zalewski M, Hallquist MN, et al: Developmental trajectories of borderline personality disorder symptoms and psychosocial functioning in adolescence. J Pers Disord 30(3):351–372, 2016b 26067158

Yen S, Peters JR, Nishar S, et al: Association of borderline personality disorder criteria with suicide attempts: findings from the collaborative longitudinal study of personality disorders over 10 years of follow-up. JAMA Psychiatry 78(2):187–194, 2021 33206138

Young JE, Klosko J, Weishaar ME: Schema Therapy: A Practitioner's Guide. New York, Guilford Press, 2003

Yuodelis-Flores C, Ries RK: Addiction and suicide: a review. Am J Addict 24(2):98–104, 2015 25644860

Zanarini MC, Frankenburg FR: A preliminary, randomized trial of psychoeducation for women with borderline personality disorder. J Pers Disord 22(3):284–290, 2008 18540800

Zanarini MC, Gunderson JG, Frankenburg FR, Chauncey DL: Discriminating borderline personality disorder from other axis II disorders. Am J Psychiatry 147(2):161–167, 1990 2301653

Zanarini MC, Vujanovic AA, Parachini EA, et al: A screening measure for BPD: the McLean Screening Instrument for Borderline Personality Disorder (MSI-BPD). J Pers Disord 17(6):568–573, 2003 14744082

Zanarini MC, Frankenburg FR, Hennen J, et al: Axis I comorbidity in patients with borderline personality disorder: 6-year follow-up and prediction of time to remission. Am J Psychiatry 161(11):2108–2114, 2004 15514413

Zanarini MC, Weingeroff JL, Frankenburg FR: Defense mechanisms associated with borderline personality disorder. J Pers Disord 23(2):113–121, 2009b 19379090

Zanarini MC, Frankenburg FR, Weingeroff JL, et al: The course of substance use disorders in patients with borderline personality disorder and Axis II comparison subjects: a 10-year follow-up study. Addiction 106(2):342–348, 2011a 21083831

Zanarini MC, Horwood J, Wolke D, et al: Prevalence of DSM-IV borderline personality disorder in two community samples: 6,330 English 11-year-olds and 34,653 American adults. J Pers Disord 25(5):607–619, 2011b 22023298

Zanarini MC, Frankenburg FR, Reich DB, et al: Attainment and stability of sustained symptomatic remission and recovery among patients with borderline personality disorder and axis II comparison subjects: a 16-year prospective follow-up study. Am J Psychiatry 169(5):476–483, 2012 22737693

Zanarini MC, Weingeroff JL, Frankenburg FR, Fitzmaurice GM: Development of the self-report version of the Zanarini rating scale for borderline personality disorder. Pers Mental Health 9(4):243–249, 2015

Zanarini MC, Conkey LC, Temes CM, Fitzmaurice GM: Randomized controlled trial of web-based psychoeducation for women with borderline personality disorder. J Clin Psychiatry 79(3):52–59, 2018 28703950

Zemore SE, Kaskutas LA: Helping, spirituality and Alcoholics Anonymous in recovery. J Stud Alcohol 65(3):383–391, 2004

Zemore SE, Kaskutas LA: 12-step involvement and peer helping in day hospital and residential programs. Subst Use Misuse 43(12–13):1882–1903, 2008 19016170

Zemore SE, Lui C, Mericle A, et al: A longitudinal study of the comparative efficacy of Women for Sobriety, LifeRing, SMART Recovery, and 12-step groups for those with AUD. J Subst Abuse Treat 88:18–26, 2018 29606223

Zielinski MJ, Veilleux JC: Examining the relation between borderline personality features and social support: the mediating role of rejection sensitivity. Pers Individ Dif 70:235–238, 2014

Zimmerman M, McGonigal P, Moon SS, et al: Does diagnosing a patient with borderline personality disorder negatively impact patient satisfaction with the initial diagnostic evaluation? Ann Clin Psychiatry 30(3):215–219, 2018 30028896

Zlotnick C, Donaldson D, Spirito A, Pearlstein T: Affect regulation and suicide attempts in adolescent inpatients. J Am Acad Child Adolesc Psychiatry 36(6):793–798, 1997 9183134

Zywiak WH, Longabaugh R, Wirtz PW: Decomposing the relationships between pretreatment social network characteristics and alcohol treatment outcome. J Stud Alcohol 63(1):114–121, 2002 11925053

A Summary of Research Trials on Evidence-Based Treatments for Alcohol/ Substance Use Disorder and Borderline Personality Disorder

Julia Jurist, B.A.
Sam Mermin, B.A.
Georgia Steigerwald
Lois Choi-Kain, M.D., M.Ed.
Hilary Connery, M.D., Ph.D.

Dynamic Deconstructive Psychotherapy

Dynamic deconstructive psychotherapy (DDP) is a psychodynamic psychotherapy that integrates translational neuroscience and object relations theory to treat individuals with borderline personality disorder (BPD) combined with co-occurring substance use disorders (SUDs). DDP facilitates the emotion processing central to all psychotherapies, which both alcohol use and borderline personality neurocognitive features impede. DDP also instructs clinicians to pay attention to splitting as manifested through denial and shame systems, which patients use defensively so that in the short run they feel relief from anxiety but in the long run interfere with their management of reality. Treatment involves individual weekly sessions for 12 to 18 months, established in the treatment plan. Adjunctive treatment including medications and groups are encouraged but not required.

Dialectical Behavior Therapy

Dialectical behavior therapy (DBT) is a treatment originally developed for suicidal patients who did not respond to usual cognitive-behavioral therapy techniques. These suicidal treatment nonresponsive patients tended to meet criteria for BPD. Linehan thereby founded the first treatment that was scientifically effective for patients with BPD by adding a dialectical attitude combining accepting validation of the patient's problems at hand with a push for change to do better and find more effective solutions for problems of emotional dysregulation that drive self-destructive behaviors. DBT has been adapted as a treatment for co-occurring SUDs (Dimeff and Linehan 2008), but this variant is not published in a full manual format nor has that adaptation been adequately trialed. DBT aims to balance strategies for acceptance or validation of emotional states with strategies for behavioral change. Standard DBT consists of individual psychotherapy, skills groups, and individual skills coaching sessions. Targets for behavioral change are conceptualized hierarchically, with suicidal and treatment-interfering behaviors representing the top of the hierarchy. Adaptations of DBT for SUDs apply this same combination of emotional validation and attempt at behavioral change to patients' substance use, and incorporate increasing days abstinent and sober mindedness as a primary targets. Some adaptations of DBT for co-occurring SUDs include medication to treat SUDs.

Dual-Focused Schema Therapy

Dual-focused schema therapy (DFST) combines behavioral and symptom-focused skills for relapse prevention with an exploration of the schemas that patients developed early in life for understanding themselves, others, and their environments. DFST is based on the theory that altering a small number of consequential, maladaptive schemas can have an enormous influence on the behaviors and interpersonal interactions that are causing both substance use and personality dysfunction. DFST is an individual therapy originally designed to be delivered over 24 weeks.

Table A–1. Comparative features of treatments

Treatment	Model	Intensity (h/wk)	Duration (months)	Modalities	Focus	Managing safety
DBT	Emotional dysregulation	~3–4	12	Individual, group, medications	Tolerating and regulating emotions and acting skillfully	Phone coaching around the clock
DDP	Impaired neurocognition and splitting	~1–2	12–18	Individual	Emotion processing, denial, and shame systems	Exploration of antecedents of suicidal or self-injurious wishes; high threshold for hospitalization
DFST	Maladaptive schemas	~1–2	6	Individual	Cognition	Safety contracting; contingencies for suicide/ self-injury; exploration of pros and cons of suicidal/ self-injurious behavior
GPM	Interpersonal hypersensitivity	~1–2	12	Individual, group, and family therapy with medication as needed	Symptomatic states and social transactions	Determined by setting and realistic availability; safety plan

DBT = dialectical behavior therapy; DDP = dynamic deconstructive therapy; DFST = dual-focus schema therapy; GPM = good psychiatric management.

Table A–2.   Research trials on DBT for BPD and AUD/SUD

Reference	Inclusion criteria	Groups and sample characteristics	Interventions	Outcome variables and measurement points	Findings
Linehan et al. 1999	BPD SUD	DBT (*n*=12) TAU (*n*=15) Mean age=30.4	DBT: 1 hour weekly individual therapy; 2 hours (plus 15-minute wind down) weekly skills training group; skills coaching phone consultation as needed; weekly team meetings of all therapists TAU: Referred to alternate treatment in the community for SUD, BPD, or both, or continued with existing psychotherapy if already in treatment	Drug use: Proportion of days abstinent from alcohol/ drugs BPD symptoms: Parasuicide History Interview, Social Adjustment Scale (scores include Global Adjustment Scale, Global Social Adjustment), State-Trait Anger Expression Inventory Longitudinal Interview Follow-Up Evaluation Base Schedule Assessments at pretreatment, 4, 8, 12, and 16 months	DBT > TAU proportion of days abstinent from drugs (at 4 months, 8 months, 16 months) DBT > TAU global functioning (GSA scores at 16 months) DBT > TAU social functioning (GSA scores at 16 months) DBT = TAU amount of medical and inpatient psychiatric treatments received

Table A–2. Research trials on DBT for BPD and AUD/SUD *(continued)*

Reference	Inclusion criteria	Groups and sample characteristics	Interventions	Outcome variables and measurement points	Findings
van den Bosch et al. 2002	BPD in outpatient psychiatry or substance use disorder treatment	DBT (*n*=27) TAU (*n*=31) Female only Mean age=37.5 BPD+SUD (*n*=15) BPD without SUD (*n*=43)	DBT: weekly individual psychotherapy; 2–2.5-hour weekly skills groups; phone consultation as needed; weekly team meeting for therapists TAU (not defined)	Substance abuse: Addiction Severity Index (European version), number of days of substance use in past month BPD symptoms: frequency of self-mutilating behavior, frequency of self-damaging impulsive acts Assessment at 12 months and 18 months	DBT = TAU days ≥ 5 drinks past month DBT = TAU days alcohol problems past month DBT = TAU days drug problems past month DBT = TAU severity alcohol problems DBT > TAU rate of retention in therapy DBT > TAU reduction of self-mutilating behavior DBT > TAU reduction of self-damaging impulsive acts Presence of substance abuse did not impact efficacy of DBT on BPD symptomatology

Table A–2.   Research trials on DBT for BPD and AUD/SUD *(continued)*

Reference	Inclusion criteria	Groups and sample characteristics	Interventions	Outcome variables and measurement points	Findings
Harned et al. 2008	BPD and at least 2 suicide attempts and/or NSSI acts in past 5 years	DBT (*N*=52) CBTE (*N*=49) Female only Mean age=29 AUD (*n*=8)	CBTE: Treatment from therapists nominated by community mental health leaders as experts in treatment of difficult patients. Therapists who self-identified as cognitive or behavioral in orientation were excluded. Condition was developed to control for various measures of treatment quality	Substance dependence: drug- and alcohol-free days, time meeting remission criteria from DSM-IV Assessment weekly throughout 1 year of treatment and 1 additional year of follow-up assessment	DBT > CBTE proportion of days abstinent from drugs and alcohol during treatment DBT > CBTE proportion of days abstinent from drugs and alcohol at follow-up DBT > CBTE full remission from SDD DBT > CBTE time spent in partial remission from SDD

AUD=alcohol use disorder; BPD=borderline personality disorder; CBTE=enhanced cognitive-behavioral therapy; DBT=dialectical behavior therapy; GAS=Global Assessment Scale; SDD=substance dependence disorder; SUD=substance use disorder; TAU=treatment as usual.

Table A–3. Research trials on DDP for BPD and AUD/SUD

Reference	Inclusion criteria	Groups and sample characteristics	Interventions	Outcome variables and measurement points	Findings
Gregory et al. 2008	BPD, and alcohol abuse or dependence	DDP (*n*=15) TAU (*n*=15) Mean age=28.7	DDP: Weekly, manualized, individual psychotherapy for 12–18 month duration. Encouraged to engage in group therapy as well, medication management in line with APA guidelines for BPD. TAU: Referral to an alcohol rehabilitation center, list of clinics and providers who may be able to provide treatment, patients in treatment allowed to keep current therapist (most subjects received individual psychotherapy and medication management).	Parasuicide behavior: Lifetime parasuicide count (adapted 3-month version) Alcohol misuse: Addiction severity index Institutional care: Days spent in inpatient psychiatric unit, inpatient detoxification/ rehabilitation facility, emergency department, partial hospitalization program, group home, halfway house Assessments at intake, 3 months, 6 months, 12 months	DDP > TAU parasuicidal episodes DDP > TAU alcohol misuse DDP > TAU institutional care use reduction

Table A-3. Research trials on DDP for BPD and AUD/SUD *(continued)*

Reference	Inclusion criteria	Groups and sample characteristics	Interventions	Outcome variables and measurement points	Findings
Gregory et al. 2010	Same as above (follow-up study with participants who completed original study and responded to contact)	DDP (*n*=8) TAU (*n*=8) Sample	Same as above (follow-up study)	Borderline symptom change: Borderline Evaluation of Severity Over Time Drinking behavior: Addiction Severity Index Assessment at 30 months from original enrollment (18 months from conclusion of original study)	DDP > TAU BPD symptom reduction DDP > TAU heavy drinking behavior reduction (non-significant effect)

APA = American Psychiatric Association; BPD = borderline personality disorder; DDP = dynamic deconstructive therapy; TAU = treatment as usual.

Table A–4. Research trials on DFST for BPD and AUD or SUD

Reference	Inclusion criteria	Groups and sample characteristics	Interventions	Outcome variables and measurement points	Findings
Ball et al. 2011	BPD and referred for residential treatment with external pressures from State of Connecticut institutions.	DFST (*n*=12) IDC (*n*=19)	DFST: 2 months individual psychotherapy focused on addiction coping skills and education about personality schemas, relationships, coping; 4 months focused on change strategies IDC: Psychotherapy focused exclusively on addiction	Symptom change: Brief Symptom Inventory of psychiatric symptoms, Inventory of Interpersonal Problems, Multiple Affect Adjective Checklist (for dysphoria) Assessment monthly for 6 months	DFST = IDC symptom reduction during first 3 months of treatment DFST < IDC symptom reduction months 3–6

BPD = borderline personality disorder; DFST = dual-focus schema therapy; IDC = individualized drug therapy.

Table A–5. Research trials on GPM for BPD and AUD/SUD

Reference	Inclusion criteria	Groups and sample characteristics	Interventions	Outcome variables and measurement points	Findings
McMain et al. 2009	BPD and suicidal behavior or non-suicidal self-injury 9.4% current SUD 59% lifetime SUD	DBT (*n*=90) GPM (*n*=90) 86% female Mean age=30.36	DBT: weekly individual psychotherapy (1 hour); weekly skills groups (2 hours); phone coaching (2 hours); weekly team meeting for therapists TAU: One hour weekly psychodynamically informed therapy; symptom-targeted medication management; weekly therapist supervision	Suicide and self-injury: suicidal and self-injurious episodes Health care utilization: emergency department visits, emergency department visits for suicidal behavior, days in psychiatric hospital BPD symptoms: Zanarini Rating Scale for BPD, Beck Depression Inventory, State-Trait Anger Expression Inventory, Symptom Checklist for symptom distress, Inventory of Interpersonal Problems Assessments at baseline, 4 months, 8 months, 12 months	GPM = DBT suicide attempts, non-suicidal self-injury, health care utilization, borderline symptoms, depression, interpersonal functioning, symptom distress, anger

Table A–5. Research trials on GPM for BPD and AUD/SUD (*continued*)

Reference	Inclusion criteria	Groups and sample characteristics	Interventions	Outcome variables and measurement points	Findings
McMain et al. 2012	Same as above (follow-up study)	Same as above	Same as above	Outcome variables same as above Assessments at 18 months, 24 months, 30 months, 36 months	GPM = DBT suicide attempts, non-suicidal self-injury, health care utilization, borderline symptoms, depression, interpersonal functioning, symptom distress, anger
Wnuk et al. 2013	Same as above (follow-up study)	Same as above	Same as above	Treatment dropout: Failure to attend four consecutive scheduled treatment sessions	GPM > DBT treatment retention for patients with greater Axis I co-occurrence

Table A–5. Research trials on GPM for BPD and AUD/SUD (continued)

Reference	Inclusion criteria	Groups and sample characteristics	Interventions	Outcome variables and measurement points	Findings
Penzenstadler et al. 2018	BPD patients in a single treatment arm 41% AUD 52% any SUD	BPD without SUD (n=48) BPD with SUD (n=51)	GPM: 10 sessions weekly individual outpatient therapy, augmented for some participants by the MOTR. Groups combined for analysis.	BPD symptoms: Outcome Questionnaire 45.2, Borderline Symptom list Therapeutic alliance: Working Alliance Inventory (Short form)	BPD + SUD = BPD without SUD borderline symptom improvement BPD + SUD > BPD without SUD increase in therapeutic alliance over time

AUD=alcohol use disorder; BPD=borderline personality disorder; DBT=dialectical behavior therapy; GPM=good psychiatric management; MOTR=motive-oriented therapeutic relationship; SUD=substance use disorder; TAU=treatment as usual.

B

General Psychiatric Management Toolkit

General Psychiatric Management Adherence Scale

The General Psychiatric Management Adherence Scale (GPMAS; Kolla et al. 2009) assesses adherence by monitoring key clinical tasks that constitute good care for patients with borderline personality disorder (BPD), rating 48 items on a scale of 1 (no emphasis) to 5 (major emphasis) during the prior session. GPMAS uses an overall mean score as well as subscale scores. In a trial of 10-session general psychiatric management (Kolly et al. 2016), adherence measured by this instrument explained 23% variance in the improvement of BPD symptoms and 16% related to improvement of general symptoms. GPMAS serves additionally as an organizing checklist for clinicians to monitor their comprehensive coverage of good management procedures for patients with BPD. See the end of this section.

Harvard Medical School Continuing Medical Education Online Course on General Psychiatric Management

- Website: https://pll.harvard.edu/course/general-psychiatric-management-bpd
- The 8-hour McLean Gunderson Personality Disorders Institute course teaches mental health professionals what they need to know to become competent providers who can derive satisfaction from treating

these patients. Through lectures, case vignettes, and interactive decision points, the course covers management strategies such as practicality, good sense, and flexibility. It describes techniques and interventions that facilitate the patient's trust and willingness to become a proactive collaborator. It reviews guidelines for managing the common and usually most burdensome issues of managing suicidality and self-harm (e.g., intersession crises, threats as a call for help, excessive use of emergency departments or hospitals). Furthermore, it describes how and when psychiatrists can usefully integrate group, family, or other psychotherapies.

- Date: Available until September 25, 2025
- Cost: $45
- Provided by: Harvard Medical School Continuing Medical Education; Gunderson Personality Disorders Institute at McLean Hospital
- Length: 8 hours
- Continuing Medical Education (CME) credits provided for physicians, nurse practitioners, registered nurses, physician assistants, psychologists, social workers, licensed mental health counselors.

Table B–1. General Psychiatric Management Adherence Scale (Kolla et al. 2009)

Item	1 Not at all	2	3	4	5 Completely present
Subscale 1: Assessment procedures					
1. Completing safety evaluation					
2. Determining treatment setting or level of care required					
3. Assessing for presence of comorbid disorders					
4. Assessing functional impairments, needs, and goals					
5. Examining intrapsychic conflicts and defenses					
6. Examining development progress and arrests					
7. Examining adaptive and maladaptive coping styles					
8. Examining psychosocial stressors					
9. Examining strengths					
10. Determining other concurrent treatments needed					
Subscale 2: Establishing treatment contract					
11. Establishing the treatment framework					
12. Determining readiness for psychotherapy					
13. Encouraging concurrent treatments					
14. Identifying ongoing care providers					
15. Developing crisis management plan					

Table B-1. General Psychiatric Management Adherence Scale (Kolla et al. 2009) (*continued*)

Item	1 Not at all	2	3	4	5 Completely present
Subscale 3: Ongoing case management					
16. Responding to crises and safety monitoring					
17. Establishing a therapeutic framework and alliance					
18. Maintaining a therapeutic framework and alliance					
19. Providing education about the disorder and its treatment					
20. Coordinating the treatment effort					
21. Monitoring and reassessing clinical status and treatment plan					
22. Encouraging multimodal treatment					
23. Intervening regarding functioning					
Subscale 4: General principles of psychotherapy					
24. Some form of psychotherapy offered					
25. Demonstrating flexibility					
26. Attending to role of patient preference in terms of the focus of the psychotherapy					
27. Dealing with setting boundaries					
28. Conducting skills training					
29. Demonstrating empathy and validation					
30. Conveying feasible expectations					

Table B-1. General Psychiatric Management Adherence Scale (Kolla et al. 2009) *(continued)*

Item	1 Not at all	2	3	4	5 Completely present
31. Set up expectations for responsible behavior					
32. Let positive transference alone					
33. Active with early signs of negative transference					
Subscale 5: Focus on feelings					
34. Focusing on identification of feelings					
35. Commenting about facial expressions					
36. Remarking on body language					
37. Clarifying maladaptive responses to feelings					
38. Connecting behaviors to events or thoughts or feelings					
39. Inquiring whether anything new has been learned					
40. Fostering clients' interest or curiosity					
41. Using clients' words and language					
Subscale 6: Specific therapeutic issues					
42. Taking a rehabilitation focus					
43. Expanding the focus away from self-harm					
44. Visiting early trauma in session					
45. Exploring body image distortion					

Table B-1.　General Psychiatric Management Adherence Scale (Kolla et al. 2009) *(continued)*

Item	1 Not at all	2	3	4	5 Completely present
46. Expecting or encouraging competitiveness					
47. Discussing intersession contacts					
48. Discussing termination					

Source. Kolla NJ, Links PS, McMain S, et al: Demonstrating adherence to guidelines for the treatment of patients with borderline personality disorder. Can J Psychiatry 54(3):181–189, 2009 19321022. Reprinted by permission of SAGE Publications.

C

Guidelines for Families

Goals: Go Slowly

1. Remember that change is difficult to achieve, and the prospect of it is fraught with fear. Be cautious about suggesting that "great" progress has been made or giving "you can do it" reassurances. "Progress" evokes fears of abandonment.
2. Lower your expectations. Set realistic goals that are available. Solve big problems in small steps. Work on one thing at a time. "Big" goals or long-term goals lead to discouragement and failure.

Family Environment: Keep Things Cool

1. Keep things cool and calm. Appreciation is normal. Tone it down. Disagreement is normal. Tone it down, too.
2. Maintain family routines as much as possible. Stay in touch with family and friends. There's more to life than problems, so don't give up the good times.
3. Find time to talk. Chats about light or neutral matters are helpful. Schedule times for this if you need to.

Managing Crises: Pay Attention But Stay Calm

1. Don't get defensive in the face of accusations and criticisms. However unfair these may be, say little and don't fight. Allow yourself to be hurt. Admit to whatever is true in the criticisms.
2. Self-destructive acts or threats require attention. Don't ignore them. Don't panic. Don't keep secrets about this. Talk about it openly with your family member and make sure professionals know.

3. Listen. People need to have their negative feelings heard. Don't say "it isn't so." Don't try to make their feelings go away. Using words to express fear, loneliness, inadequacy, anger, or needs is good. It is better to use words than to act on feelings.

Addressing Problems: Collaborate and Be Consistent

1. When solving a family member's problems, ALWAYS
   a. Involve the family member in identifying what needs to be done.
   b. Ask whether the person can "do" what is needed in the solution.
   c. Ask whether the person wants you to help them "do" what is needed.

2. Family members need to act in concert with one another. Parental inconsistencies fuel severe family conflicts. Develop strategies that everyone can stick to.

3. If you have concerns about medications or therapist interventions, make sure that both your family member and their therapist or doctor know. If you have financial responsibility, you have the right to address your concerns to the therapist or doctor.

Limit Setting: Be Direct But Careful

1. Set limits by stating the limits of your tolerance. Let your expectations be known in clear, simple language. Everyone needs to know what is expected of them.

2. Do not protect family members from the natural consequences of their actions. Allow them to learn about reality. Bumping into a few walls is usually necessary.

3. Do not tolerate abusive treatment such as tantrums, threats, hitting, and spitting. Walk away and return to discuss the issue later.

4. Be cautious about using threats and ultimatums. They are a last resort. Do not use threats and ultimatums as a means of convincing others to change. Present them only when you can and will carry through. Let others—including professionals—help you decide when to give them.

Adapted from Gunderson and Links 2014.

D

Online Resources for Borderline Personality Disorder and Alcohol Use Disorder

Julia Jurist, B.A.
Sam Mermin, B.A.
Georgia Steigerwald
Lois Choi-Kain, M.D., M.Ed.
Hilary Connery, M.D., Ph.D.

Adapted from Choi-Kain and Gunderson 2019 and Harrison and Connery 2019.

General Resources for Consumers, Families, and Clinicians

988 Suicide and Crisis Lifeline

Call: 9–8–8
Information: https://www.samhsa.gov/find-help/988

American Foundation for Suicide Prevention

https://afsp.org

National Alliance on Mental Illness (NAMI)

http://www.nami.org

Research on Alcoholism

www.niaaa.nih.gov

Borderline Personality Disorder

National Education Alliance for Borderline Personality Disorder (NEABPD)

- https://www.borderlinepersonalitydisorder.com/
- Information—provides information about BPD for patients, families, Family Connections leaders, and professionals; also includes information on GAP (Global Alliance for Prevention and Early Intervention for BPD) and a podcast. The Family Guidelines are provided in various languages.
- Links—to national organizations, research and treatment
- Referral source—none; has a "Looking for Treatment" page with suggestions on finding the right treatment and professional
- Lists—recommends publications, books, a library of articles, and the NEABPD journal; a media library including conference presentation and course/workshop videos

McLean Hospital Borderline Personality Disorder Family and Consumer Education

- Initiative—webinar series by BPD experts at McLean Hospital
- Videos for all audiences—Webinars include Common Questions About Borderline Personality Disorder and What You Can Do To Help; How Can I Recognize Borderline Personality Disorder? (conducted in Spanish); Difficult Conversations: How to Discuss Borderline Personality Disorder With a Loved One; General Psychiatric Management (GPM) for the Treatment of Borderline Personality Disorder; Family Struggles and Strategies to Address Common Challenges; The Coexistence of Borderline Personality Disorder and Substance Misuse (https://www.mcleanhospital.org/video/coexistence-borderline-personality-disorder-and-substance-misuse)

Project Air (Australia)

- **https://www.projectairstrategy.org/**
- Fact Sheets—Provide resources relevant to patients, families, schools, and clinicians. For patients, answer useful and relevant questions such as "You've been diagnosed with BPD, what now?" Offer relatable useful facts, self-help resources, and parenting tools for those with BPD. For clinicians, offers basic toolkit of pragmatic guidance.
- Adolescent Brief Intervention Manual for Complex Mental Health Issues—A brief (four-session) intervention centered around creating a Care Plan for the young person and a Support Plan for their carer. May be useful as a stepping-stone before longer term care.

Borderline Personality Disorder Support Services in South Australia

- **http://bpdsa.com.au/**
- Website—Provides information for consumers, carers, and clinicians. For consumers and carers, there are several links to helpful websites such as Project Air and SANE Australia. There are also resources for finding care for individuals living in Australia. For clinicians, there are links to relevant research, websites, and some in-person and online training options.
- Online Library—Also provides a link to free online library of research and resources regarding how clinicians can best work with families and carers. The contents of the library include videos, training manuals, and empirical research articles.

BPD Foundation

- **https://www.bpdfoundation.org.au/**
- Website—Psychoeducational materials on BPD, its coexisting disorders, and its treatments, including books, presentations and conferences, and research articles
- Lists—Online resources for people with BPD, their carers, and general practitioners.
- Additional resources on help tips, recovery, and multicultural mental health.
- Resources for Consumers and Their Families

National Alliance on Mental Illness (NAMI)

- http://www.nami.org
- Information—Find BPD under the topic "About Mental Illness" (click on "Mental Health Conditions" and then "Borderline Personality Disorder). Provides information about etiology, comorbidities, treatment, self-harm, and medications.
- Links—Information on treatment modalities for BPD, "A BPD Brief" (Gunderson 2006), substance use disorders, self-injury, family connection reading list, and mental illnesses discussion groups. Additionally, a link to the National Education Alliance for Borderline Personality Disorder and National Institute of Mental Health websites.
- Referral source—For state and local affiliates that provide support, education, information, referral, and advocacy

Emotions Matter

- https://emotionsmatterbpd.org/
- What Is BPD?—Factual information on prevalence, the disorder itself (neurobiology, symptoms, etc.), common misconceptions, and treatment.
- Programs—Online peer support groups, social connections, Facebook group, advocacy efforts.
- Resources—Access to downloadable guides for students with BPD and those affected by self-harm for the student, the carers, and school administrators. A list of organizations, online resources, and books.

Personality Disorder Awareness Network (PDAN)

- http://www.pdan.org/
- Information—Provides information on personality disorders, including BPD, and has a blog, online parenting programs, and recordings of past webinars.
- Links—To national and international organizations such as NAMI, NIMH, and Australian Organization for BPD.
- Referral source—Link to Theravive, a network of mental health professionals in the US and Canada, GoodTherapy.org, and PsychologyToday.com.
- Lists—Recommended books such as helpful options for children (e.g., The Weather House: Living With a Parent With Borderline Personality Disorder).

New York Presbyterian BPD Resource Center

• **https://www.nyp.org/bpdresourcecenter**
• Information—Provides information on diagnosis and treatment; instructional videos by experts regarding symptoms, treatment, and recovery; and audio recordings of individuals with BPD telling their own stories.
• Lists—Informational websites, recommended books by both experts and individuals with BPD, and publications for professionals.

SANE Australia: Guide to Borderline Personality Disorder

• **https://www.sane.org/information-stories/facts-and-guides/ borderline-personality-disorder#help-for-people-with-bpd**
• Help for people with BPD—Walks an individual with BPD through what a BPD diagnosis means, options for care, staying safe in a crisis, and getting support.
• Help for family, friends, and carers—Provides a guide for families/ friends regarding how to connect with a person with BPD, how to look out for themselves, and how to help someone in a crisis.

Resources for Clinicians

Stanley-Brown Safety Plan

• **https://suicidesafetyplan.com/**

Dynamic Deconstructive Psychotherapy (DDP)

• **Information and resources—https://www.upstate.edu/psych/ education/residency/psychotherapy/dynamic_decon.php**
• Web-based supplementary training program in DDP
• https://www.upstate.edu/psych/education/residency/ psychotherapy/ddp-training/index.php

Alcohol Use Disorder

Helplines That Provide Referrals for Treatment

U.S. Substance Abuse and Mental Health Services Administration Referral Helpline:
(800) 662–4357

The Addiction Policy Forum Alcohol and Drug Helpline:
(301) 200–3658

List of Alcoholism/Addiction Treatment Programs

List of Addiction Treatment Programs by ZIP Code
   https://findtreatment.gov/

National Institute on Alcohol Abuse and Alcoholism Treatment Navigation Tool
   https://alcoholtreatment.niaaa.nih.gov/how-to-find-alcohol-treatment/
step-1-search-trusted-sources-to-find-providers

Accredited Rehab Facilities
   https://www.carf.org/providerSearch.aspx
   Commission on Accreditation of Rehabilitation Facilities. Use "Advanced Search" for alcoholism, alcohol use, etc.

State-Funded Rehab Programs
   To find out what state-funded programs are available, contact the state agency in charge of substance-abuse services. Contact information for each state agency can be found here: https://www.samhsa.gov/sites/
default/files/ssadirectory.pdf
   Information is also available via the U.S. Substance Abuse and Mental Health Services Administration Referral Helpline ((800) 662–4357) for programs that are state-funded, have a sliding-fee scale, or accept Medicare or Medicaid.

Directories of Physicians Who Specialize in Addiction Treatment

American Society of Addiction Medicine:
   https://www.asam.org/publications-resources/patient-resources/fad
American Board of Addiction Medicine:
   https://www.abam.net/find-a-physician
American Academy of Addiction Psychiatry:
   https://www.aaap.org/education/resources/patients/find-a-specialist/

National Association of Addiction Treatment Providers:
  https://www.naatp.org/resources/addiction-industry-directory

Directory of Psychologists Who Specialize in Addiction

https://locator.apa.org/ (enter "addiction" in the Provider Name search box)

List of Vivitrol (Naltrexone) Providers for Alcohol Dependence by ZIP Code
  https://www.vivitrol.com/alcohol-dependence/find-a-provider

Treatment Directories Outside of the United States

Canada

A government-funded directory of programs in Ontario:
  www.connexontario.ca/Search/AdvancedSearch

A privately run but comprehensive list of programs by province:
  www.drugrehab.ca

A directory of government-funded programs for First Nations and Inuit peoples:
  www.canada.ca/en/indigenous-services-canada/services/addictions-treatment-first-nations-inuit.html

United Kingdom

The National Health Service (NHS) offers a directory of alcohol addiction support services by location:
  https://www.nhs.uk/nhs-services/find-alcohol-addiction-support-services/

Public Health England offers a rehab directory:
  www.rehab-online.org.uk

A directory of treatment services in Scotland:
  https://www.scottishdrugservices.com/

Ireland

A searchable directory of addiction services:
  www.services.drugs.ie

A list of addiction services provided by the Health Service Executive:
www.hse.ie/eng/services/list/5/addiction

An alcoholism helpline run by the Health Service Executive:
1800 459 459

Australia

A national alcohol and drug hotline run by the Australian government can direct you to local services. The number is: 1800 250 015.

A directory of Queensland treatment providers:
www.qnada.org.au/service-finder/#

New Zealand

A national alcohol and drug helpline can be contacted at: 0800 787 797.

A list of additional resources provided by the Mental Health Education and Resource Centre:
www.mherc.org.nz/directory/alcohol-drug-other-addiction-services

Support Groups

Alcoholics Anonymous

- Main website —https://www.aa.org/
- To find meetings by location—https://www.aa.org/find-aa
- Online meetings—https://aa-intergroup.org/

Dual Recovery Anonymous (for people with an addiction and emotional or psychiatric illness)

- Main website—https://draonline.org/
- To find meetings—https://draonline.org/meetings/

Secular AA (online AA-type meetings without religious content)

- https://www.aasecular.org/

Celebrate Recovery (Christ-centered Twelve-Step program)

- Main website—https://www.celebraterecovery.com/
- Meetings—https://locator.crgroups.info/

In the Rooms (online-only meetings)

- https://www.intherooms.com/home/

SMART Recovery (nonreligious group using behavioral principles to address a wide variety of addiction issues)

- Main website—www.smartrecovery.org
- Meetings in the United States and Canada—www.smartrecovery-test.org/local
- Meetings in the United Kingdom—https://smartrecovery.org.uk/online-meetings/
- Meetings in Australia—https://smartrecoveryaustralia.com.au/

Women for Sobriety (female-only group for alcoholics and drug users)

- Main website—www.womenforsobriety.org
- Meetings in the US and Canada—www.womenforsobriety.org/meetings

Secular Organizations for Sobriety

- Main website—www.sossobriety.org
- Meetings—www.sossobriety.org/find-a-meeting

LifeRing Secular Recovery

- Main website—www.lifering.org
- Meetings in the US—https://lifering.org/f2f-meetings/
- Online meetings—https://lifering.org/f2f-meetings/
- International meetings—https://lifering.org/f2f-meetings/international-meetings/

Moderation Management (reducing harm from drinking rather than strict abstinence)

- Main website—www.moderation.org
- Meetings—https://moderation.org/events/

Recovery Dharma (based on Buddhist teachings, peer-led, abstinence-based)

- Main website—https://recoverydharma.org
- Meetings—https://recoverydharma.org/meetings/

Refuge Recovery (based on Buddhist teachings, peer-led, abstinence based)

- Main website—https://www.refugerecovery.org/
- Meetings—https://refugerecoverymeetings.org/meetings

For Families

Substance Abuse and Mental Health Services Administration (SAMHSA)

- https://www.samhsa.gov/families

CRAFT (Community Reinforcement and Family Training)

Coaching from another parent:

- Helpline of the Partnership for Drug-Free Kids: (855) 378–4373

Books:

- Beyond Addiction: How Science and Kindness Help People Change (Foote et al. 2014)
- Get Your Loved One Sober: Alternatives to Nagging, Pleading, and Threatening (Meyers and Wolfe 2009)
- The Parent's 20 Minute Guide, Second Edition, and The Partner's 20 Minute Guide, Second Edition (Center for Motivation and Change 2016a, 2016b)

Al-Anon (largest support group for families of alcoholics, based on Twelve-Step principles)

- Main website—www.al-anon.org
- Meetings in the US—www.al-anon.org/al-anon-meetings/find-an-al-anon-meeting
- Meetings outside the US—www.al-anon.org/al-anon-meetings/worldwide-al-anon-contacts
- Online meetings—www.al-anon.org/al-anon-meetings/virtual-meetings

Alateen (Al-Anon for teenagers)

- Main website—www.al-anon.org/for-members/group-resources/alateen
- Meetings in the US—www.al-anon.org/al-anon-meetings/find-an-alateen-meeting
- Meetings outside the US—www.al-anon.org/al-anon-meetings/worldwide-al-anon-contacts

Families Anonymous (Twelve-Step group for families)

- Main website—www.familiesanonymous.org
- Meetings—https://familiesanonymous.org/meetings/meeting-directories/

Adult Children of Alcoholics (Twelve-Step group)

- Main website—www.adultchildren.org
- Meetings—https://adultchildren.org/meeting-search/

Searchable Directory of Family Support Groups

- www.supportgroupproject.org

Helpline Providing Support for Families

- Addiction Policy Forum: (833) 301–4357
- SMART Recovery Family and Friends
- Main website—www.smartrecovery.org/family
- Meetings—www.smartrecoverytest.org/local

Parents of Addicted Loved Ones

- Main website—www.palgroup.org
- Meetings—www.palgroup.org/find-a-meeting

Because I Love You (BILY)

- Main website—www.bily.org
- Meetings—www.bily.org/get-help/meeting-locations

Shatterproof Family Support Programs

- Main website—www.shatterproof.org/shatterproof-family-support-programs
- More information—(800) 597–2557 or info@shatterproof.org

Grief Recovery After Substance Passing (GRASP)

- Main website—www.grasphelp.org
- Meetings—www.grasphelp.org/community/meetings

For Clinicians

Motivational Interviewing

- https://motivationalinterviewing.org/

Neuroscience-Based Nomenclature (for psychopharmacology)

- https://www.ecnp.eu/research-innovation/nomenclature

Screening Instruments

Julia Jurist, B.A.
Sam Mermin, B.A.
Georgia Steigerwald
Lois Choi-Kain, M.D., M.Ed.
Hilary Connery, M.D., Ph.D.

Borderline Personality Disorder

(See next page.)

Table E-1. Borderline Symptom List 23 (BSL-23)

	Not at all	A little	Rather	Much	Very strong
In the course of last week….					
1) It was hard for me to concentrate	0	1	2	3	4
2) I felt helpless	0	1	2	3	4
3) I was absent-minded and unable to remember what I was actually doing	0	1	2	3	4
4) I felt disgust	0	1	2	3	4
5) I thought of hurting myself	0	1	2	3	4
6) I didn't trust other people	0	1	2	3	4
7) I didn't believe in my right to live	0	1	2	3	4
8) I was lonely	0	1	2	3	4
9) I experienced stressful inner tension	0	1	2	3	4
10) I had images that I was very much afraid of	0	1	2	3	4
11) I hated myself	0	1	2	3	4
12) I wanted to punish myself	0	1	2	3	4
13) I suffered from shame	0	1	2	3	4
14) My mood rapidly cycled in terms of anxiety, anger, and depression	0	1	2	3	4
15) I suffered from voices and noises from inside or outside my head	0	1	2	3	4
16) Criticism had a devastating effect on me	0	1	2	3	4
17) I felt vulnerable	0	1	2	3	4

Table E–1. Borderline Symptom List 23 (BSL-23) (*continued*)

	Not at all	A little	Rather	Much	Very strong
18) The idea of death had a certain fascination for me	0	1	2	3	4
19) Everything seemed senseless to me	0	1	2	3	4
20) I was afraid of losing control	0	1	2	3	4
21) I was disgusted by myself	0	1	2	3	4
22) I felt as if I was far away from myself	0	1	2	3	4
23) I felt worthless	0	1	2	3	4

Quality of your overall personal state in the course of the last week. 0% means absolutely down, 100% means excellent.

0%   10%   20%   30%   40%   50%   60%   70%   80%   90%   100%

↑   ↑   ↑   ↑   ↑   ↑   ↑   ↑   ↑   ↑   ↑

(very bad)   (excellent)

Table E–2. BSL – Behavior Supplement

	Not at all	Once	2–3 times	4–6 times	Daily or more often
During the last week….					
1) I hurt myself by cutting, burning, strangling, head banging, etc.	0	1	2	3	4
2) I told other people that I was going to kill myself	0	1	2	3	4
3) I tried to commit suicide	0	1	2	3	4
4) I had episodes of binge eating	0	1	2	3	4
5) I induced vomiting	0	1	2	3	4
6) I displayed high-risk behavior by knowingly driving too fast, running around on the roofs of high buildings, balancing on bridges, etc.	0	1	2	3	4
7) I got drunk	0	1	2	3	4
8) I took drugs	0	1	2	3	4
9) I took medication that had not been prescribed, or if it had been prescribed, I took more than the prescribed dose	0	1	2	3	4
10) I had outbreaks of uncontrolled anger or physically attacked others	0	1	2	3	4
11) I had uncontrollable sexual encounters of which I was later ashamed or which made me angry	0	1	2	3	4

Bohus et al. 2009

Alcohol Use Disorder

Table E–3.   CAGE Screening Tool

1.   Have you ever felt you ought to cut down on your drinking?
2.   Have people annoyed you by criticizing your drinking?
3.   Have you ever felt bad or guilty about your drinking?
4.   Have you ever had a drink first thing in the morning to steady your nerves or get rid of a hangover (eye-opener)?

"No" = 0 and "Yes" = 1. A total score of 2 or higher is considered clinically significant.

Link —https://americanaddictioncenters.org/alcoholism-treatment/cage-question-naire-assessment

Ewing 1984

AUDIT-C (Alcohol Use Disorders Identification Test-Concise)

1. How often did you have a drink containing alcohol in the past year?

    a. Never
    b. Monthly or less
    c. Two to four times a month
    d. Two to three times a week
    e. Four or more times a week

2. How many drinks did you have on a typical day when you were drinking in the past year?

    a. None, I do not drink
    b. 1 or 2
    c. 3 or 4
    d. 5 or 6
    e. 7 to 9
    f. 10 or more

3. How often did you have six or more drinks on one occasion in the past year?

    a. Never
    b. Less than monthly
    c. Monthly
    d. Weekly
    e. Daily or almost daily.

Scored 0–12 (0 reflecting no alcohol use). Score of 4 or more for men and 3 or more for women considered positive.

Bush et al. 1998

https://doi.org/10.1001/archinte.158.16.1789

AUDIT-PC (Alcohol Use Disorders Identification Test-Piccinelli Consumption)

Assessing hazardous alcohol intake in primary care setting.

1. How often did you have a drink containing alcohol in the past year?

    a. Never
    b. Monthly or less
    c. Two to four times a month
    d. Two to three times a week
    e. Four or more times a week

2. How many drinks did you have on a typical day when you were drinking in the past year?

    a. None, I do not drink
    b. 1 or 2
    c. 3 or 4
    d. 5 or 6
    e. 7 to 9
    f. 10 or more

3. How often during the last year have you found that you were not able to stop drinking once you had started?

    a. Never
    b. Less than monthly
    c. Monthly
    d. Weekly
    e. Daily or almost daily

4. How often during the last year have you failed to do what was normally expected from you because of drinking?

    a. Never
    b. Less than monthly
    c. Monthly
    d. Weekly
    e. Daily or almost daily

5. Has a relative, friend, doctor or other health worker been concerned about your drinking or suggested you should cut down?

   a. Never
   b. Yes, but not in the last year
   c. Yes, during the last year

Score of 4 or more as a cutoff.
Piccinelli et al. 1997

Clinical Institute Withdrawal Assessment-Alcohol, Revised (CIWA-Ar)

1. **Nausea/vomiting:** Do you feel sick to your stomach? Have you vomited?

     0—no nausea and no vomiting
     1—mild nausea with no vomiting
     2
     3
     4—intermittent nausea with dry heaves
     5
     6
     7—constant nausea, frequent dry heaves and vomiting

2. **Tremor:** Extend arms and spread fingers apart. Observe…

     0—no tremor
     1—not visible, but can be felt fingertip to fingertip
     2
     3
     4—moderate, with patient's arms extended
     5
     6
     7—severe, even with arms not extended

3. **Paroxysmal sweats:** Observe…

     0—no sweat visible
     1—barely perceptible sweating, palms moist
     2
     3
     4—beads of sweat obvious on forehead
     5
     6
     7—drenching sweats

4. **Anxiety:** Do you feel nervous? Observe...

> 0—no anxiety, at ease
> 1—mildly anxious
> 2
> 3
> 4—moderately anxious, or guarded, so anxiety is inferred
> 5
> 6
> 7—equivalent to acute panic states as seen in severe delirium or acute schizophrenic reactions

5. **Agitation:** Observe...

> 0—normal activity
> 1—somewhat more than normal activity
> 2
> 3
> 4—moderately fidgety and restless
> 5
> 6
> 7—paces back and forth during most of the interview, or constantly thrashes about

6. **Tactile disturbances:** Have you any itching, pins and needles sensations, any burning, any numbness, or do you feel bugs crawling on or under your skin?

> 0—none
> 1—very mild itching, pins and needles, burning or numbness
> 2—mild itching, pins and needles, burning or numbness
> 3—moderate itching, pins and needles, burning or numbness
> 4—moderately severe hallucinations
> 5—severe hallucinations
> 6—extremely severe hallucinations
> 7—continuous hallucinations

7. **Auditory disturbances:** Are you more aware of sounds around you? Are they harsh? Do they frighten you? Are you hearing anything that is disturbing to you? Are you hearing things you know are not there?

> 0—not present
> 1—very mild harshness or ability to frighten
> 2—mild harshness or ability to frighten
> 3—moderate harshness or ability to frighten

4—moderately severe hallucinations
5—severe hallucinations
6—extremely severe hallucinations
7—continuous hallucinations

8. **Visual disturbances:** Does the light appear to be too bright? Is its color different? Does it hurt your eyes? Are you seeing anything that is disturbing to you? Are you seeing things you know are not there?

0—not present
1—very mild sensitivity
2—mild sensitivity
3—moderate sensitivity
4—moderately severe hallucinations
5—severe hallucinations
6—extremely severe hallucinations
7—continuous hallucinations

9. **Headache, fullness in head:** Does your head feel different? Does it feel like there is a band around your head? Do not rate for dizziness or lightheadedness. Otherwise, rate severity.

0—not present
1—very mild
2—mild
3—moderate
4—moderately severe
5—severe
6—very severe
7—extremely severe

10. **Orientation and clouding of sensorium:** What day is this? Where are you? Who am I?

0—oriented and can do serial additions
1—cannot do serial additions or is uncertain about date
2—disoriented for date by no more than 2 calendar days
3—disoriented for date by more than 2 calendar days
4—disoriented for place and/or person

Maximum score of 67. Pharmacological treatment potentially indicated for score of 10 or more, use clinical judgment for scores of 10 to 20.
Sullivan et al. 1989

Short Alcohol Withdrawal Scale (SAWS)

	None (0)	Mild (1)	Moderate (2)	Severe (3)
Anxious				
Sleep disturbance				
Problems with memory				
Nausea				
Restless				
Tremor (shakes)				
Feeling confused				
Sweating				
Miserable				
Heart pounding				

Scores of 12 or above suggested as likely to require medication to reduce withdrawal severity and increase probability of treatment retention.
Gossop et al. 2002

Addiction Severity Index – single question

1. In the past month, how many days have you had 5 or more drinks containing alcohol (wine, beer, liquor, etc.)?

McLellan et al. 1992

American Society of Addiction Medicine Patient Placement Criteria (ASAM-PPC)

-   0.5 Early Intervention
-   Level 1 Outpatient Services
-   Level 2.1 Intense Outpatient Services
-   Level 2.5 Partial Hospitalization Services
-   Level 3.1 Clinically Managed Low-Intensity Residential Services
-   Level 3.3 Clinically Managed Population-Specific High-Intensity Residential Services
-   Level 3.5 Clinically Managed High-Intensity Residential Services

- Level 3.7 Medically Monitored Intensive Inpatient Services
- Level 4 Medically Managed Intensive Inpatient Services

   Within each of these levels, patients are considered on six dimensions and given severity rankings which are from 0 (no issue) to 4 (highest risk/ imminent danger).

- Dimension 1 (Acute intoxication and/or withdrawal potential)
- Dimension 2 (Biomedical conditions and complications)
- Dimension 3 (Emotional, behavioral, or cognitive conditions and complications)
- Dimension 4 (Readiness for change)
- Dimension 5 (Relapse, continued use or continued problem potential)
- Dimension 6 (Recovery/living environment)

   Hoffman 1993

Index

Page numbers printed in **boldface** type refer to figures, boxes, and tables.